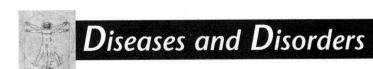

Diseases and Disorders

Cystic Fibrosis

Titles in the Diseases and Disorders series include:

Alzheimer's Disease
Anorexia and Bulimia
Arthritis
Asthma
Attention Deficit Disorder
Autism
Breast Cancer
Chronic Fatigue Syndrome
Cystic Fibrosis
Diabetes
Down Syndrome
Epilepsy
Hemophilia
Hepatitis
Learning Disabilities
Leukemia
Lyme Disease
Multiple Sclerosis
Phobias
Schizophrenia
Sleep Disorders
Small Pox

Diseases and Disorders

Cystic Fibrosis

by Melissa Abramovitz

LUCENT BOOKS®

THOMSON
GALE

San Diego • Detroit • New York • San Francisco • Cleveland
New Haven, Conn. • Waterville, Maine • London • Munich

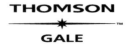

THOMSON

━━━━━✳━━━━━™

GALE

On Cover: A young cystic fibrosis patient receives physiotherapy.

LIBRARY OF CONGRESS CATALOGING-IN-PUBLICATION DATA

Abramovitz, Melissa, 1954
    Cystic fibrosis / by Melissa Abramovitz.
        p. cm. — (Diseases and disorders)
    Summary: Explores the history, symptoms, diagnosis, and treatment of cystic
fibrosis, reviews ongoing research, and discusses how to live with the incurable
genetic disease that is often called "65 Roses."
    Includes bibliographical references and index.
    ISBN 1-59018-299-5 (hc: alk. paper)
    1. Cystic fibrosis—Juvenile literature. [1. Cystic fibrosis. 2. Diseases.]
    I.Title. II. Diseases and disorders series.
    RC858.C95 A274 2003
    616.3'7—dc21   2002152876

Printed in the United States of America

Table of Contents

"The Most Difficult Puzzles Ever Devised"

CHARLES BEST, ONE of the pioneers in the search for a cure for diabetes, once explained what it is about medical research that intrigued him so. "It's not just the gratification of knowing one is helping people," he confided, "although that probably is a more heroic and selfless motivation. Those feelings may enter in, but truly, what I find best is the feeling of going toe to toe with nature, of trying to solve the most difficult puzzles ever devised. The answers are there somewhere, those keys that will solve the puzzle and make the patient well. But how will those keys be found?"

Since the dawn of civilization, nothing has so puzzled people—and often frightened them, as well—as the onset of illness in a body or mind that had seemed healthy before. A seizure, the inability of a heart to pump, the sudden deterioration of muscle tone in a small child—being unable to reverse such conditions or even to understand why they occur was unspeakably frustrating to healers. Even before there were names for such conditions, even before they were understood at all, each was a reminder of how complex the human body was, and how vulnerable.

While our grappling with understanding diseases has been frustrating at times, it has also provided some of humankind's most heroic accomplishments. Alexander Fleming's accidental discovery in 1928 of a mold that could be turned into penicillin has resulted in the saving of untold millions of lives. The isolation of the enzyme insulin has reversed what was once a death sentence for anyone with diabetes. There have been great strides in combating conditions for which there is not yet a cure, too. Medicines can help AIDS patients live longer, diagnostic tools such as mammography and ultrasounds can help doctors find tumors while they are treatable, and laser surgery techniques have made the most intricate, minute operations routine.

This "toe-to-toe" competition with diseases and disorders is even more remarkable when seen in a historical continuum. An astonishing amount of progress has been made in a very short time. Just two hundred years ago, the existence of germs as a cause of some diseases was unknown. In fact, it was less than 150 years ago that a British surgeon named Joseph Lister had difficulty persuading his fellow doctors that washing their hands before delivering a baby might increase the chances of a healthy delivery (especially if they had just attended to a diseased patient)!

Each book in Lucent's *Diseases and Disorders* series explores a disease or disorder and the knowledge that has been accumulated (or discarded) by doctors through the years. Each book also examines the tools used for pinpointing a diagnosis, as well as the various means that are used to treat or cure a disease. Finally, new ideas are presented—techniques or medicines that may be on the horizon.

Frustration and disappointment are still part of medicine, for not every disease or condition can be cured or prevented. But the limitations of knowledge are being pushed outward constantly; the "most difficult puzzles ever devised" are finding challengers every day.

No Longer Just a Childhood Disease

C YSTIC FIBROSIS, ALSO known as CF, used to be considered solely a childhood disease. That is because people born with the disorder rarely survived past their childhood years. Indeed, says the Cystic Fibrosis Foundation, "When the CF Foundation was founded in 1955, a child with CF was not expected to live much beyond the age of five."[1]

Besides being fatal to many babies and children, cystic fibrosis remained a mysterious ailment that no one understood for many years. Even the name cystic fibrosis was a confusing and difficult-to-pronounce symbol of adversity. While medical experts were unable to ease the hardship of living with CF until the last decade of the twentieth century, the Cystic Fibrosis Foundation relates a touching story of how one of the many small children who had the disease in 1965 came up with a nickname that a kid could at least pronounce. Four-year-old Richard Weiss, one of three brothers with CF, was listening to his mother, Mary, making phone calls to raise funds for cystic fibrosis research. As detailed on the Cystic Fibrosis Foundation website: "After several calls, Richard came into the room and told his Mom, 'I know what you are working for.' Mary was dumbstruck because Richard did not know what she was doing, nor did he know that he had cystic fibrosis. With some trepidation, Mary posed the question, 'What am I working for, Richard?' 'You are working for 65 Roses,' he answered so sweetly."[2]

Since that time, many children with CF have referred to their disease as 65 Roses, and the rose, an ancient symbol of love, has become the symbol of the Cystic Fibrosis Foundation. Having a more palatable nickname, however, did not lengthen the short life span of the children born with cystic fibrosis. Only the dedication of tireless volunteers like Mary Weiss and the ongoing efforts of doctors and researchers committed to understanding and treating the disease gradually improved the situation over the next few decades. Step by step, investigators discovered the causes of CF and developed new treatments that began to extend

A young patient with cystic fibrosis receives therapy to help clear her lungs.

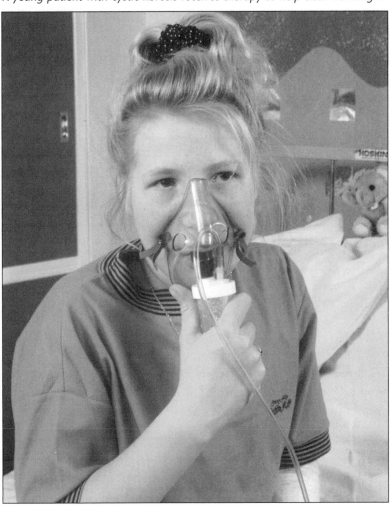

the lives of affected children. CF treatment centers were set up throughout the world, and the median survival age went from age five to age sixteen in 1970, age eighteen in 1980, age twenty-nine in 1990, and age thirty-two in 2000.

Adults Now Have CF, Too

Today, many people with CF lead productive lives into their twenties, thirties, forties, and beyond. Although most of the thirty thousand Americans who currently have CF are still children, about eleven thousand adults in the United States now have the disorder. The average survival age stands at thirty-two, but more and more patients are entering their fourth, fifth, and sixth decades of life. The oldest known person with CF is over seventy.

Experts believe that the average survival time will continue to increase as more and more people receive treatment early in life, before irreversible damage takes place. And yes, even many adults with CF call the disease 65 Roses as a tribute to the remarkable progress that has occurred during their lifetime.

But even with all this progress, cystic fibrosis is still not curable, and it continues to prematurely end the lives of many children, teens, and adults throughout the world. It remains the most common lethal genetic disease among Caucasians in the United States; about one in three thousand Caucasians, one in fifteen thousand African Americans, and one in one hundred thousand Asian Americans will get CF and eventually die from it. The battle to conquer this devastating illness is far from over, and experts and affected families agree that there is still a long way to go before people with CF can look forward to a normal life span and future. In a *Philadelphia Inquirer* article, Roland Merullo, whose daughter has CF, expressed the overwhelming aura of fatality that surrounds those who live with the disease:

> Everyone associated with cystic fibrosis senses the shadow of premature death hovering around the edges of every conversation on the subject. . . . One visits a CF clinic and sees two unusually thin teenagers sitting close beside their mother in the

waiting room, not mixing with the other kids, their faces revealing a seriousness beyond their years and the sense that college, marriage, and a career are things to dream about, rather than plan for.[3]

Although a cure will never come soon enough for those who daily face the prospect of a life cut short by CF, the efforts of many doctors, nurses, researchers, volunteers, and other dedicated individuals bring hope and optimism each day. A plethora of laboratory experiments and clinical trials continues to improve the quality of life for the thousands of babies, children, and adults who presently have cystic fibrosis, and for the first time in history, scientists now know what is required to achieve a cure. No one knows how long it will be until such a cure is perfected, but the outlook for CF patients looks brighter each and every day.

Chapter 1

What Is Cystic Fibrosis?

S CIENTISTS BELIEVE CYSTIC fibrosis has affected humans for over fifty thousand years. Anthropologists who have studied people's migration patterns throughout history believe the disease originated in the Middle East. As people from this region migrated to other areas, CF went with them until it appeared in virtually every civilization on the planet. Although CF is not contagious, it is transmitted through a person's genes, and at the present time it is known to strike every racial and ethnic group to some extent. Caucasians, however, remain the group most frequently affected.

Although CF has been around for a long time, no one recognized its many symptoms as being part of a single medical disorder until the mid-twentieth century. The most prominent symptom that people referred to before the 1900s was the characteristic salty tasting skin of children who had a mysterious, as yet unnamed ailment. "Woe is the child who tastes salty from a kiss on the brow, for he is hexed, and soon must die,"[4] states a quote from the Middle Ages, when the first recorded reference to a CF-like disease surfaced.

The Mysterious Disease Gets a Name

Aside from these early descriptions of the salty skin of children with this unnamed disease, not much was written about it until around 1900, when several physicians described a disorder of newborn infants in which the baby was unable to properly digest food and had chronic lung infections. It was not until 1938, however, that doctors realized these symptoms were related to a single disease process.

In 1938 Dr. Dorothy Anderson of Columbia University in New York published the first description of cystic fibrosis as a distinct illness. Anderson studied many case histories of infants and children with a combination of breathing and digestive problems. She also performed autopsies on children who had died from the condition. Upon finding scars in the digestive organ called the pancreas and infection and damage in the lungs, Anderson realized that the digestive and respiratory symptoms were part of a single disorder. She chose the name cystic fibrosis of the pancreas because fluid-filled pockets, or cysts, were surrounded by patches of fibrous scar tissue. The name was later shortened to cystic fibrosis.

Soon afterward, other doctors discovered that children with the disease had thick, sticky mucus clogging the ducts in certain glands and in body organs like the lungs and pancreas. In 1952 a severe summer heat wave in New York City provided physicians with still another clue about the defining characteristics of CF. A large number of children with the disease were admitted to area hospitals with severe dehydration. Dr. Paul di Sant-Agnese and his associates at the Columbia University College of Physicians and Surgeons discovered that the reason for the dehydration was that these children were losing abnormally large amounts of salt in their sweat. Although the doctors did not know why this was happening, their observations put experts on the right track toward understanding that the salty sweat and thick, sticky mucus were hallmark qualities of CF that could help explain the entire disease process.

Doctors now know that cystic fibrosis is primarily characterized by the abnormal flow of ions (charged particles) of sodium and chloride, the elements in salt, in cells that line the lungs, pancreas, intestines, liver, and exocrine glands. Exocrine glands secrete chemicals through ducts rather than directly into the bloodstream through cell walls. Examples include sweat and reproductive glands.

A defect in the process by which sodium and chloride ions normally cross cell membranes is responsible for the abnormal ion flow. The defect does not allow chloride channels, the tiny gates through which these chemicals move, to open. This results in large quantities of thick, sticky mucus, which block the normal function of these organs and glands, leading to the characteristic symptoms and complications of the disease. The other primary characteristic seen in cystic fibrosis, overly salty sweat, is produced because excessive amounts of sodium chloride are expelled from the sweat glands onto the skin's surface.

A physician treats an infant afflicted with CF. The baby's body is plagued with the presence of thick mucus, a hallmark of CF.

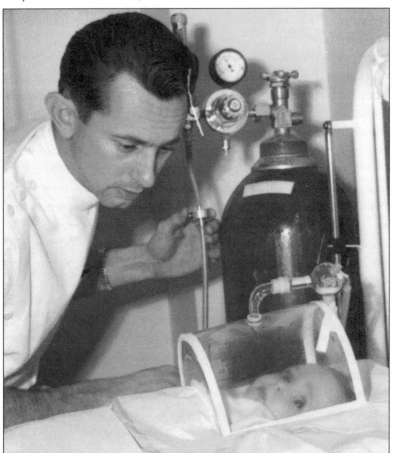

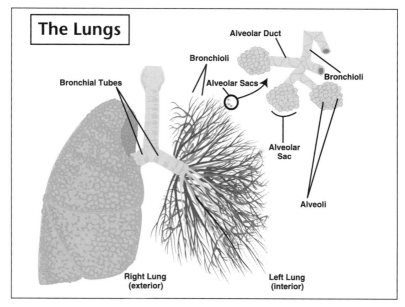

The Lungs

Alveolar Duct
Bronchioli
Bronchial Tubes
Alveolar Sacs
Bronchioli
Alveolar Sac
Alveoli
Right Lung (exterior)
Left Lung (interior)

Although the same underlying malfunction is responsible for the different problems associated with each affected organ or gland system, the actual symptoms, of course, depend on the designated purpose and function of the specific body part.

How CF Affects the Lungs

The job of the lungs and respiratory system, also referred to as the pulmonary system, is to bring oxygen into the body and to expel carbon dioxide. Air is inhaled through the nose or mouth, then goes through the trachea, or windpipe, into the bronchi, where it is filtered, warmed, and humidified. The bronchi consist of several levels of branching tubes that lead into the lungs. After traveling through these tubes, air ends up in tiny sacs known as alveoli. Alveoli look like little balloons that inflate and deflate with each breath. They are surrounded by small blood vessels called capillaries. When air inflates the alveoli, oxygen from the air passes through the thin cell walls and enters the capillaries. From these tiny blood vessels, oxygen penetrates the bloodstream, where red blood cells carry this life-giving gas to all the body tissues. The red blood cells also carry carbon dioxide waste products from these tissues back to the lungs. There, the alveoli take on the carbon dioxide and release it back through the branching bronchi. Finally, the carbon dioxide is exhaled through the nose or mouth.

In addition to playing a role in taking in air and breathing out carbon dioxide, the bronchial airways also secrete mucus to keep the lungs moist and to trap bacteria and other particles. The cells that make this mucus are known as epithelial cells; they line the walls of the airways. Also lining these walls are tiny hairlike brushes called cilia. Cilia push trapped bacteria and other pollutants upward so they can be expelled with a sneeze or cough.

Respiratory Complications from Cystic Fibrosis

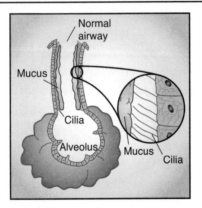

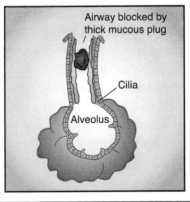

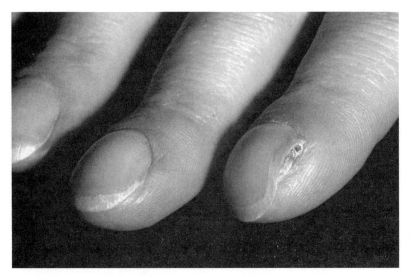

These fingernails exhibit clubbing, a common side effect of the lung infections that CF patients experience.

With cystic fibrosis, the mucus produced by the epithelial cells is too thick and sticky to be cleared out efficiently. The small airways become blocked, and then the lungs cannot process oxygen and carbon dioxide in a normal manner. If not corrected, this complication can lead to respiratory failure, a potentially fatal condition in which the blood oxygen levels fall too low and carbon dioxide levels are too high. The blockage can also induce heart disease from the strain of having to pump more oxygen-bearing blood to the narrowed airways.

Other common respiratory complications from CF are asthma, in which the bronchial muscles tighten and the airways become inflamed, leading to breathing difficulties; sinusitis, an irritation of the sinus cavities in the head; and nose polyps, or small growths in the nose that result from breathing problems and sometimes make them worse. Atelectasis, in which a completely blocked airway leaves part of the lung with no air; emphysema, in which air becomes trapped in the alveoli; and pneumothorax, a collapsed lung that results from air bursting from the alveoli and deflating the lung, are also frequently seen complications.

The most common lung problem that CF patients experience is chronic obstructive pulmonary disease (COPD). The thick mucus blocks and inflames the airways, leading to coughing, wheezing, and a high risk of lung infections. Bacteria, viruses, and occasionally fungi are responsible for the infections that COPD triggers, with bacteria being the usual culprit. Depending on where the resulting infection lodges, the illness may be referred to as bronchitis or pneumonia. Bronchitis affects the bronchial tubes, while pneumonia usually means the infection is somewhere in the lungs besides the bronchi.

Most people with CF become infected by the bacteria *Staphylococcus aureus*, *Pseudomonas aeruginosa*, or *Burkholderia cepacia* at some time during the course of their illness. If the infections are not eradicated, a vicious cycle of inflammation and progressive lung damage may result. The white blood cells the immune system sends to fight the infection die and release their DNA (deoxyribonucleic acid) into the mucus, making it even stickier. The body will also naturally produce more mucus to try to flush out the infection, and this further blocks the airways and leads to more breathing problems. Another common complication from chronic lung infections is clubbing, which appears when chemicals the body makes to try to contain the infection cause the tissue at the base of the fingernails and toenails to swell. It is respiratory failure, however, that claims the lives of about 95 percent of cystic fibrosis patients.

The Digestive System and CF

Another body system that is usually affected by cystic fibrosis is digestion. The main job of the digestive system is to bring food into the body, process it, and eliminate waste. After food enters through the mouth, it proceeds down the esophagus to the stomach, where hydrochloric acid and pepsin begin to digest it. The partly digested food then goes to the small intestine; it is here that digestion is completed, usable nutrients are released into the bloodstream, and waste is passed along to be excreted.

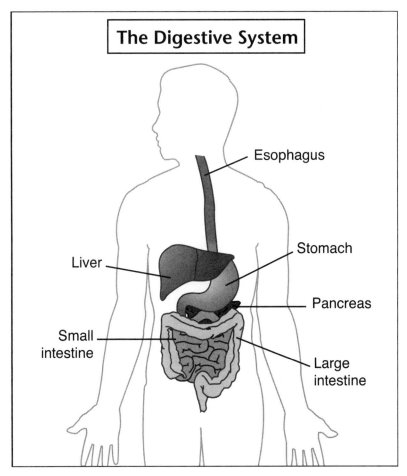

The Digestive System

Esophagus

Stomach

Liver

Pancreas

Small intestine

Large intestine

The small intestine secretes some digestive enzymes of its own, but it cannot do its job without help from the liver and pancreas. The liver releases bile, which helps digest fats, into the intestine through bile ducts. The pancreas supplies several enzymes including trypsin, chymotrypsin, and lipase. Pancreatic enzymes are made by cells called acini, which send these products through pancreatic ducts into the intestine. Each enzyme is responsible for breaking down different types of food, primarily proteins and fats. The pancreas also produces insulin, a hormone that is not actually involved in digestion but is responsible for allowing glucose, the energy source for cells throughout the body, to enter these cells.

In cystic fibrosis, cells lining the liver and pancreatic ducts produce large amounts of thick, sticky mucus, which block the flow of enzymes from the pancreas and bile from the liver. The buildup of enzymes in the pancreas creates small growths known as cysts; these become surrounded by scar tissue that eventually destroys the pancreas. These cysts and fibrous scars were in fact the basis for the name cystic fibrosis. If the scar tissue destroys certain all-important cells that produce insulin, diabetes may result. About 40 percent of CF patients who live to adulthood end up with diabetes from the progressive damage to the pancreas.

In addition, since the pancreatic enzymes cannot get to the small intestine because of the mucous plugs, nutrients like proteins and fats are not completely digested and are expelled as waste matter. This can lead to malnourishment, even if the person consumes an adequate amount of food. One of the hallmark symptoms of CF is a good appetite but poor weight gain due to the body not absorbing enough nutrients. Related symptoms may include a bloated abdomen and an overall weakness, which may in turn worsen the lung infections seen in people with CF.

Because each drop of a CF patient's sweat (pictured, center) is excessively salty, patients must guard against the danger of dehydration during hot weather.

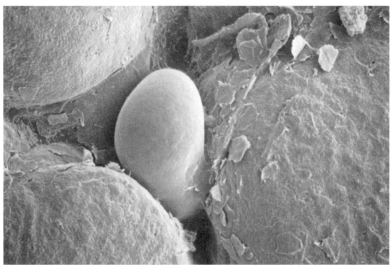

Along with causing malnutrition, the lack of pancreatic enzymes also leads to bulky, fatty stools, abdominal pain, and even intestinal blockages. Sometimes these intestinal blockages, known as meconium ileus in newborns, occur before a baby is born and must be removed immediately after birth to prevent serious complications. This happens in 5 to 10 percent of babies with CF. In rare instances, the blockage causes the intestine to burst before the baby is even born. Rebecca's mother, for example, was nine months pregnant when her unborn child experienced a ruptured intestine. Several surgeries were required to repair the problem immediately after birth. Fortunately, the little girl survived this potentially fatal complication.

In the liver, bile duct blockages from mucous plugs can also cause problems, though such effects are seen less frequently than are those involving the pancreas. Five to 10 percent of CF patients get cirrhosis, a condition in which scar tissue prevents the liver from performing its many functions, which include storing nutrients and purifying poisons and waste products in addition to aiding digestion. Mucous plugs can also result in jaundice: When bile duct blockages prevent the drainage of wastes from dead red blood cells, the skin takes on the yellowish tinge characteristic of this condition.

Sweat Glands and CF

One exocrine gland system that CF seriously impacts is the sweat glands. These glands help the body get rid of some waste products and regulate body temperature. Most people produce between one pint and one-half gallon of sweat each day. The sweat contains mostly sodium and chloride and some calcium and potassium.

Humans have over 2 million sweat glands. They reside in the skin's outermost layer, the epidermis, and each coiled sweat gland duct would measure over four feet if it were uncoiled. Thus, each person's body contains about six miles of sweat ducts.

Sweat normally moves from the base of the sweat gland through these ducts to the skin's surface. Passages known as chloride ion channels line these ducts and normally reabsorb chloride after sweat leaves the body. But with cystic fibrosis, chloride ions cannot pass normally through the cell membranes and end up being left on the skin's surface. Sodium also tends to leave these cells more quickly than normal, and these factors make the sweat saltier than it is in people who do not have CF. The excessive loss of salt places CF patients at high risk for dehydration and heatstroke in hot weather or after vigorous exercise.

The Impact of CF on the Reproductive System

The other exocrine gland system that CF most usually affects is the reproductive system. In men, the reproductive glands in the testicles are responsible for manufacturing sperm to be delivered to the penis via the vas deferens tube. In women, the main function of the reproductive system is to dispense eggs from the ovaries; these eggs then travel through the Fallopian tubes and may be fertilized at the base of the uterus. The sex hormones, which become active at puberty, initiate these processes in both men and women.

Males and females with CF generally produce normal sex hormones and thus experience sexual maturation during adolescence. Often this maturation is somewhat delayed due to general growth and health issues, but it usually happens eventually. However, most individuals with CF are infertile because of the thick mucus blocking the reproductive ducts. In men, the vas deferens tube is either blocked by mucus or completely degenerates from mucous plugs accumulated before birth, making 98 percent of males with the disease infertile. With women, mucus around the cervix at the base of the uterus blocks sperm from entering, thereby inhibiting fertilization. Some females with CF do manage to get pregnant, but many cannot.

Symptoms and Diagnosis

Although most people with cystic fibrosis experience symptoms relating to the lungs, pancreas, sweat glands, and reproductive system, the severity and onset of these symptoms vary widely. Even though everyone who has CF is born with the disease, some individuals develop life-threatening symptoms in infancy, while others are only mildly affected for many years and may not suspect that something serious is wrong. In addition, many of the symptoms of CF are similar to those seen in other diseases. "Because most of the symptoms are not unique to CF and may be somewhat mild, doctors sometimes fail to diagnose the disease in infants,"[5] explains Karen Hopkin, the author of *Understanding Cystic Fibrosis*.

All of these factors can make diagnosing CF a difficult and lengthy process. Nicholas, for example, had breathing problems throughout his childhood and was initially diagnosed with asthma. But at age eight, he developed a severe case of pneumonia, and doctors ran tests that revealed CF. Shannan, whose symptoms were mild enough that she never experienced any medical emergencies, knew something was chronically wrong but was not diagnosed with cystic fibrosis until age twenty-two.

The majority of CF patients today learn what is wrong with them well before the age Shannan did; in fact, most receive a definitive diagnosis by age two or three thanks to dramatic improvements in diagnostic techniques. The first step in the diagnostic process is for the physician to analyze the patient's family history. Since CF is a genetic disorder, knowing that one person in a family has it can be an important clue. If a sibling has CF, for example, any suspicious symptoms in a brother or sister can probably be attributed to the same disease. A physical examination and several laboratory tests can then be used to confirm the diagnosis.

When there is no family history of CF, it is not as easy to get on the correct diagnostic path. A physician who believes a patient with breathing difficulties has asthma, for instance, may not suspect CF until other symptoms like poor weight gain or serious lung infections become evident.

Laboratory Tests

Several laboratory tests can help rule out or confirm a diagnosis of cystic fibrosis. In newborns suspected of having the disease, a blood test for a protein called immunoreactive trypsinogen

(IRT) can be useful, since infants with CF usually have abnormally high levels of this protein. IRT is a building block for certain pancreatic enzymes that aid digestion. However, too much IRT may also result from other disease processes, so finding an excess does not necessarily mean the baby has CF. Doctors also run genetic tests to check for abnormalities related to CF in order to confirm a preliminary diagnosis of CF based on an IRT test. Genetic tests call for the use of sophisticated techniques for separating and viewing the microscopic genes and chromosomes found in the nucleus of cells taken from the patient's blood or from the inside of the cheek.

Since genetic tests are not 100 percent accurate, a test known as the sweat test must also be done to confirm a diagnosis of CF. The sweat test was developed by Dr. Paul di Sant-Agnese and his colleagues at the Columbia University College of Physicians and Surgeons after the 1952 New York heat wave brought many dehydrated children with CF into the hospital. Based on the observation that these children's sweat was saltier than normal, di Sant-Agnese and his group devised a method of measuring the amount of chloride in a sweat sample. Lewis Gibson and Robert Cooke, two physicians at Johns Hopkins University Hospital in Baltimore, helped make the test effective by finding an efficient way of collecting sweat, and soon doctors all over the world had accepted the sweat test as a reliable method of diagnosing CF.

To perform the sweat test, a laboratory technician applies a colorless, odorless sweat-generating chemical called pilocarpine to a small area on the patient's arm or leg. An electrode is attached to the same area, and a weak electric current is used to help stimulate sweating. The technician then collects the sweat on a piece of filter paper or gauze, or in a plastic coil, and sends the specimen to a laboratory for analysis.

Normal children have under forty millimoles of chloride per liter of sweat. A millimole is a measurement of the concentration of a particular chemical in a certain amount of liquid. Kids with CF may have two to five times the normal level of chloride. Sixty millimoles of chloride per liter of fluid is sufficient for a diagnosis of CF. Some people with the disease have much more chloride than this in their sweat, but doctors point out that higher levels do not necessarily predict a more severe case of CF. Some people with extremely high chloride levels have very mild symptoms, and, conversely, some with lower chloride levels may exhibit severe symptoms and complications.

Experts consider the sweat test to be the most accurate diagnostic test available for CF. "The Sweat Test has been the 'gold standard' for diagnosing cystic fibrosis (CF) for more than 40 years. When it is performed by trained technicians and evaluated in an experienced, reliable laboratory, the Sweat Test is still the best test to diagnose CF,"[6] explains the Cystic Fibrosis Foundation. Nevertheless, the sweat test does not work well on infants, who do not have active sweat glands yet, and thus the IRT and genetic tests are considered to be the best methods of making a diagnosis in a baby.

Another test that is very accurate for diagnosing CF is rarely used because few hospitals and laboratories have the expertise to handle it. The procedure, known as the nasal PD (potential difference) test, was developed in the 1980s after several groups of researchers discovered that people with CF had elevated electrical charges in the cells affected by their disease. "This test is probably even better than the sweat test in separating those with CF from those without," says Dr. David M. Orenstein in *Cystic Fibrosis: A Guide for Patient and Family*. "The problem with it is that it is very difficult to do correctly, and very few centers are set up to do this testing."[7]

The Importance of Early Diagnosis

With reliable diagnostic tests like the sweat test widely available, doctors are able to diagnose most people with CF at a young age. This is important, because much of the organ damage CF produces accumulates over the years, and early detection means that treatment to slow this damage can be started immediately. Anyone born with CF will have it for life, but receiving an accurate diagnosis as early as possible means that the affected individual has a greater chance of managing the disease successfully for many years.

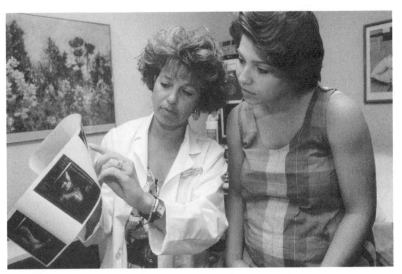

A doctor reviews prenatal test results to determine whether her patient's baby has cystic fibrosis.

With the availability of modern techniques of screening for genetic diseases before a baby is even born, many people with a family history of CF are electing to have prenatal testing so treatment can be initiated right after the birth of an affected baby. Studies have shown that "children diagnosed by screening demonstrated improved survival, a greater increase in body weight, and a slower decline in FEVI [a measurement of lung function] over the first twelve years of life. Analysis of CF patient data has shown that children whose CF is detected at birth experience fewer hospitalizations, fewer illnesses, and better nutritional status during the first two years of life."[8]

Improved diagnostic techniques are only part of the reason that more and more people with CF are now living longer and healthier lives. Along with these advances has come subsequent progress in understanding the causes of the disorder and in using this knowledge to implement successful treatment strategies.

Chapter 2

What Causes Cystic Fibrosis?

ALTHOUGH DOCTORS BEGAN making headway into effectively diagnosing cystic fibrosis in the 1940s and 1950s, it was not until the late 1980s that anyone understood what actually caused the disease. Prior to this time, experts postulated that some sort of mysterious "CF factor" produced the symptoms and complications, but no one ever defined or explained what this factor was. Experts also observed that the disorder occurred more often in certain families and thus probably had a genetic basis, but this causative element also remained a mystery until the late 1980s.

These sweat gland cells produce saltier sweat for those with CF; similar defects in epithelial cells in the lungs produce a more serious mucus buildup.

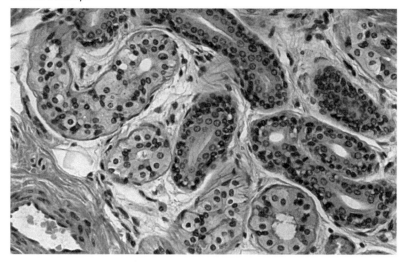

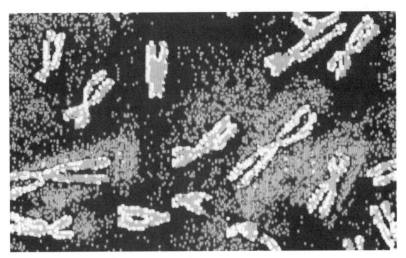

Chromosomes (pictured) contain a DNA sequence that determines which traits, including diseases like cystic fibrosis, may be inherited.

Dr. Paul Quinton at the University of California, Riverside, conducted some of the pioneering research into uncovering the causes of cystic fibrosis. Quinton discovered that the epithelial cells that line sweat gland ducts do not absorb chloride in people with the disease. Normally, these epithelial cells take up chloride from the sweat that flows from the base of the sweat gland to the skin's surface. But with CF, the chloride cannot get through the cell membrane. The negatively charged chloride ions also pull along positively charged sodium ions, and both the sodium and chloride build up in the sweat, producing its characteristic saltiness.

Other studies in the 1980s revealed that the epithelial cells in the lungs of people with CF had similar defects. Michael Knowles and Richard Boucherat, physicians at the University of North Carolina in Chapel Hill, for instance, found that the epithelial cells lining the airways in patients' lungs were also unable to move chloride ions across their membranes. While this defect resulted in salty sweat when it occurred in the sweat glands, the outcome in the lungs was the production of the hallmark thick, sticky mucus due to the abnormal sodium chloride balance depleting the normal moisture content.

It's in the Genes

Discovering that the same defect could explain the diverse symptoms of cystic fibrosis led scientists to begin a search for the source of the defect. As medical science advanced to the point where doctors understood how the genetic material in each cell encodes instructions for the cells' operations, investigators realized that the logical place to look for the underlying cause of CF was in the genes.

Genes are the parts of a DNA molecule that pass hereditary information from parents to their offspring. They reside on wormlike bodies called chromosomes in the center, or nucleus, of each cell. The sequence of genes on each chromosome provides the cell containing those chromosomes with a set of instructions on how to grow and operate. A baby is born with two copies of this instruction set—one from each parent.

Humans have forty-six chromosomes in each cell. Twenty-three come from the mother and the other twenty-three from the father. The genes on each chromosome also come in pairs, with one copy of every gene from the mother and one from the father.

When a gene or chromosome is damaged, the resulting change is called a mutation. The damage that produces a mutation can involve an entire chromosome, one or more genes, or one or more of the chemicals that make up DNA. A DNA molecule is composed of two strands of chemical compounds known as nucleotides, which include the bases adenine, thymine, guanine, and cytosine. These strands are twisted together so that adenine is always paired with thymine and guanine with cytosine. The exact sequence of nucleotides determines the instructions encoded by a particular gene. Damage or absence of even one nucleotide is sometimes enough to totally disrupt the instructions associated with the gene.

Mutated genetic material can be passed to a child if it happens to be part of the set of chromosomes and genes transmitted from either the mother or father. When this occurs, the altered genetic instructions may cause various malfunctions that produce certain diseases or disorders.

Scientists searching for the cause of cystic fibrosis realized that a gene mutation was probably responsible for faulty instructions that resulted in the abnormally sluggish movement of chloride ions across cell membranes, and they began the arduous task of trying to find out what and where the mutation was.

The Search for the Faulty Gene Begins

Finding the gene responsible for CF was not an easy task. Searching for a tiny particle with electron microscopes and chemicals that separate DNA strands is never easy, but sometimes a genetic defect is very obvious and not too difficult to spot for experts who know what to look for. The mutation that causes one type of leukemia, for example, consists of an easily detected break in a certain chromosome. In contrast, the mutation that underlies cystic fibrosis is very difficult to detect. Rather than involving a broken chromosome, this mutation results from an error in the

The structure of DNA, which is found in our genes, is pictured in this illustration. Damaged genes can be passed on to offspring, producing diseases such as CF.

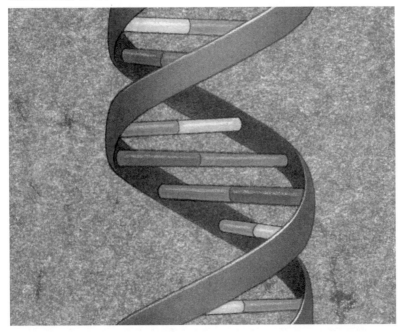

placement of only a few DNA bases, making it extremely difficult to track down. Given this fact, scientists had to employ methods that enabled them to search for specific genes on each chromosome. This way, the researchers reasoned, they could narrow the field and identify which chromosome held the gene in question.

In the early 1980s Dr. Lap-Chee Tsui and his team at the Toronto Hospital for Sick Children used a technique called linkage analysis to look for the correct chromosome. This procedure is based on the finding that genes lying close together on a chromosome tend to be inherited as a unit. Thus, the researchers looked for certain sequences of DNA that appear in the cells of families and individuals who have cystic fibrosis. These sequences are known as genetic markers. By looking for genetic markers associated with cystic fibrosis, the researchers theorized, they would eventually be able to find the chromosome that housed the faulty gene that caused the disease.

In 1985 Dr. Tsui, along with researchers from two other laboratories, published their findings that the genetic markers for CF appeared on chromosome number seven. Locating the correct chromosome was an important step toward understanding the genetic cause of the disease. "Up to that point, looking for the CF gene had been much like trying to find a particular house without even knowing what continent it was on. Now researchers could narrow their search to an area equivalent to a particular country,"[9] explain experts at the Howard Hughes Medical Institute.

The next step was to study DNA from people with and without CF to further narrow down where the critical gene was located relative to the genetic markers. But the process of painstakingly checking each DNA fragment to see whether it contained the gene was a monumental task that Dr. Tsui estimated would take about eighteen years. So he and his associates developed a method of looking for additional markers to speed up the process. They began examining thousands of samples of chromosome seven DNA to try to locate more genetic markers that would bring them closer to the elusive gene.

Tsui contacted Dr. Francis Collins at the University of Michigan to find out about Collins's new technique for analyzing one hundred thousand to two hundred thousand DNA molecules at a time. Collins called the technique "jumping," since it enabled scientists to jump, rather than walk slowly, along a chromosome searching for certain genes. Jumping involves cutting up the DNA with chemicals designed for this purpose. Then, the researchers label one end of the sliced DNA and allow the segment to curl into a circle. This puts the labeled end close to a previously noncontiguous section of DNA that ordinarily might have been thousands of bases away. The scientists can then jump quickly from one contiguous section to the other, searching for known genetic markers.

The Search Accelerates

Tsui's team collaborated with Dr. Collins and began employing the jumping technique to speed up their search. They also collaborated with Dr. John Riordan at the Toronto Hospital for

CF is caused by a genetic mutation; symptoms include the presence of thick mucus (center) in the lungs, a hallmark of CF.

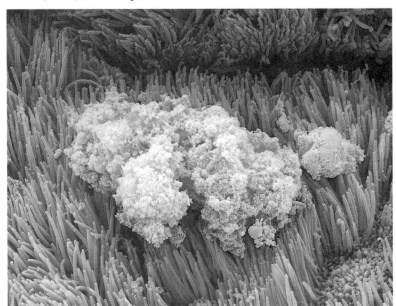

Sick Children, who was doing experiments on DNA sequences that appear in many animals. These patterns, known as conserved sequences, encode the same proteins in many species and have not changed over tens of thousands of years of evolution. They are therefore useful in matching certain genetic markers to biological functions that appear in different animals.

Riordan discovered that part of a conserved sequence on chromosome seven matched a DNA sequence that occurs in human sweat gland cells. Since doctors had already established that sweat gland epithelial cells were involved in CF, this clue brought the researchers even closer to finding the gene that causes the disease.

Tsui's team then stepped up their efforts to search for mutations in the DNA sequence they had isolated. In 1989 they found a mutation present in 70 percent of the chromosomes of people with CF. The mutation was absent in the chromosomes of people who did not have CF. Tsui, Collins, Riordan, and their colleagues had finally discovered the cystic fibrosis gene.

Later, other researchers would find that other, less frequent mutations of this very gene could also cause CF; this is why the mutation that Tsui and his colleagues discovered only occurred in 70 percent of CF patients.

The CFTR Gene

The researchers went on to show how and why the newly discovered gene was responsible for cystic fibrosis. They found that the gene issues instructions for making a certain protein they called cystic fibrosis transmembrane conductance regulator, or CFTR. This protein is essential for setting up the chloride ion channels that enable the cell to move sodium chloride across the cell membrane. A tiny error in the sequence of DNA nucleotides making up the gene—an error in which only 3 of the base pairs out of about 250,000 that make up the DNA molecule are missing—was enough to completely distort these instructions. The epithelial cells of a person with this set of garbled instructions cannot manufacture a normal CFTR protein, and therefore the normal flow of chloride ions is inhibited or entirely prevented.

CFTR is most active in the epithelial cells that line the exocrine glands, the lungs, the pancreas, and the liver. That is why cystic fibrosis primarily affects these cells. When the CFTR protein is absent or abnormal, these cells cannot regulate the flow of chloride and sodium ions in and out of the membranes, and then the cells cannot properly adjust the consistency of the fluids they secrete. Mucus secreted by the cells in these organs or glands becomes thick and sticky, resulting in mucous plugs and the subsequent symptoms of CF. Defects in sodium and chloride transport also alter the water content and cause abnormal water movement in the cells, with the result that there is not enough water to wash away all the sticky mucus.

Once scientists understood how the CF gene mutation caused the CFTR protein abnormalities, they began calling this gene the CFTR gene. Today, the acronym CFTR is used to identify both the gene that underlies CF and the protein that this gene encodes. To prevent confusion, the scientific literature uses *CFTR* for the gene and plain CFTR for the protein.

Proving the Link

In 1990 several teams of researchers presented irrefutable proof that the mutation in the CFTR gene is directly responsible for the defect in chloride transport that causes the diverse symptoms of cystic fibrosis. One team showed that they could correct the CFTR protein abnormality by inserting a normal CFTR gene into epithelial cells from the pancreas grown in a laboratory culture dish. Another group did the same thing with cells taken from the airways of the lungs.

Many experts and people affected by CF became very optimistic that this and other advances would quickly lead to a cure for the disease, but researchers found that replacing a faulty gene with a normal one was much easier to achieve in a laboratory than in a real person. After a tragic event in 1999 when a young man died after receiving a gene replacement to treat a liver disease, experiments with gene replacement in humans suffered a huge setback. New regulations were put in force, and scientists are now developing alternative methods in the hope that one day gene replacement techniques will provide a cure for CF and other devastating genetic disorders.

"The challenge has been to find a reliable way to deliver the normal genetic material to affected cells that line the airways. Several methods have been developed as delivery systems [also known as vectors], including using modified viruses, fat capsules (liposomes), and synthetic vectors. Clinical trials are under way to test the effectiveness of these delivery systems,"[10] explain doctors at the Mayo Clinic.

How Do People Get CF?

Once scientists proved that a CFTR gene mutation caused cystic fibrosis, further investigations revealed how the gene is transmitted and how different mutations of this gene are all capable of producing the disease. Genes are either dominant or recessive. As the name implies, a dominant gene overrides a recessive gene. Thus, if a child inherits a dominant gene for a particular trait from the mother and a recessive gene for the same trait from the father, the dominant trait will prevail. For example, people who are able to roll their tongue into a U shape possess the dominant gene for the trait. Only if both parents supply the recessive gene that codes for the inability to roll the tongue will a person be unable to perform a tongue roll.

The CFTR gene is a recessive gene. This means a child who develops cystic fibrosis has inherited two defective copies—one from each parent. People who inherit only one copy of the abnormal CFTR gene are called carriers. They carry the mutated gene and can pass it on to their offspring, but do not have the disease themselves. Experts estimate that over 10 million Americans carry the defective CFTR gene without actually getting the disease. Carriers have a 50 percent chance of transmitting the defective CFTR gene to a child, since each gene has a 50 percent chance of getting into an egg or a sperm cell. This means that the child of two carriers has a 25 percent chance of getting CF and a 50 percent chance of being a carrier.

Because of these high odds, many people who know they are carriers choose not to reproduce. However, many times couples are unaware of their carrier status and find out about it only after a child is born with CF. Many of these parents feel guilty, but as experts at the Mayo Clinic point out, "although parents often blame themselves when a child is born with CF, it's important to remember that nothing a parent does causes the disease."[11] Because the disease is relatively rare, these doctors say, there is no reason for people who do not know their CF carrier status to request a genetic screening test.

If one parent has CF and one is a carrier, a child has a 50 percent chance of getting the disease and a 50 percent chance of being a carrier. These odds are enough to discourage most such couples from attempting to have children. It is very unlikely that a man and a woman with CF could even conceive a baby, but if this were to happen, it is 100 percent certain that the baby would have CF.

Over a Thousand Mutations

To further complicate matters, scientists have discovered that over one thousand CFTR gene mutations are capable of causing CF. If any of these mutations is passed to an offspring by both parents, even if each parent carries a different mutation, the child will develop cystic fibrosis.

While the end result of the many CFTR mutations is the same—the disruption of chloride channels in cell membranes—the precise manner in which these mutations actually cause CF differs slightly. There are five major categories and mechanisms of action for the thousand or so CFTR mutations discovered to date.

The most common mutation, known as deltaF508, affects 70 to 80 percent of people with the disease and is an example of the first category of mutations. It causes cells to produce an abnormal CFTR protein that lacks the amino acid called phenylalanine. Amino acids are the building blocks of proteins. The *F* in deltaF508 stands for phenylalanine. The *508* indicates that phenylalanine is missing from position number 508 in the sequence of 1,480 amino acids that the CFTR protein comprises. The missing amino acid prevents the CFTR protein from folding

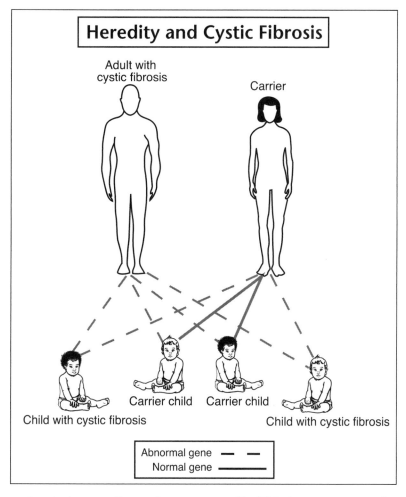

Heredity and Cystic Fibrosis

Adult with cystic fibrosis

Carrier

Carrier child   Carrier child

Child with cystic fibrosis

Child with cystic fibrosis

| Abnormal gene | — — |
| Normal gene | ——— |

and entering a cell membrane normally. This in turn causes the malfunction in chloride ion flow that underlies cystic fibrosis.

In the second major category of CFTR, gene mutations prevent the CFTR protein from being produced at all. No CFTR protein means that there is no chloride channel through which salt can be moved to the cell membrane, and this inevitably results in the symptoms of CF.

In the third type of mutation, cells produce CFTR proteins, but they are too small to function. Here the faulty gene has directed the cell to stop producing the protein before it is complete. The end result is the same as with the other types of mutations.

Mutations that cause abnormal regulation of the CFTR protein once it is made make up the fourth major category. One of the genes that carries this very rare type of mutation does allow the CFTR protein to move to the cell membrane but prevents the chloride channel from opening up. Thus, once again, the result is that the chloride cannot pass through.

The fifth and final type of mutation involves a gene that allows a complete CFTR protein to be manufactured, but because of a defective amino acid in the DNA sequence, the messages that should instruct the cell to transport chloride ions across its membrane are so garbled that this function cannot be performed correctly. Specifically, such mutations cause the chloride channels to remain open for too short a time, so barely any chloride is able to get through.

Do the Different Mutations Cause Differences in Disease Severity?

Doctors have attempted to correlate the type of gene mutation with the severity of the disease in different patients, but this line of investigation has yielded conflicting results. Most people with certain category five mutations, for example, usually have normal pancreas function, but other CF mutations do not seem to produce such consistent differences in organ function or disease severity. Thus, people with the deltaF508 mutation are more likely to experience serious ongoing lung and digestive problems, but this is not always true. Experts believe that other influences besides this gene may determine how severely the disease is manifested in a particular individual.

"Siblings, even identical twins, who possess the same CFTR mutation may not experience the same degree of severity of symptoms because of nongenetic factors, such as the environment,"[12] explains Karen Hopkin. Doctors have not yet established what these environmental influences may be, but suspect that they may involve factors in the external environment like diet and air pollution, in addition to internal biological factors.

Biologists use the phrase "genotype by environment" to characterize the process by which the internal or external environment affects how a gene works. "Genotype by environment interaction may partially explain the variation in symptoms among CF patients, even those who have exactly the same genetic mutation,"[13] say doctors writing for the Pulmonary Channel website.

One internal factor that may provide a genotype by environment influence is the presence of certain modifying genes that do not directly cause CF but seem to play a role in increasing or decreasing the intensity of symptoms. Investigators at Johns Hopkins University School of Medicine are currently trying to determine what these modifying genes may be.

A tool that scientists use to study the influence of modifying genes is genetic engineering. This involves inserting abnormal copies of the CFTR gene into developing organs of laboratory mice, thereby creating animals that have CF. Several studies have shown that some genetically engineered mice become less sick with CF if they have certain genes that activate alternative chloride channels in the lungs, pancreas, and exocrine glands. This results in less buildup of salt in the cells and less severe symptoms. Investigators are currently attempting to figure out which genes are able to activate these alternative channels. Then, they plan to test whether such modifying genes also exist in humans. Ultimately, the goal is to develop new methods of treating or even curing CF.

Chapter 3

Treatment

BEFORE DOCTORS IDENTIFIED cystic fibrosis as a specific disorder and gained an understanding of its causes, there was nothing anyone could do to treat the disease. In 1930, for example, the outlook was indeed grim for a baby born with what is now called CF, as revealed in an article in *Nurseweek*:

> When the woman gave birth to her first child, all seemed to go well at first. But within a few months she knew that something was wrong. Despite almost constant feedings, the infant was never satisfied and failed to gain weight. His bowel movements were large and bulky, and he was often inconsolable. A physician examined the infant, and a quick lick on

A young child looks out of his mist tent. Mist tents are now considered ineffective in thinning mucous production.

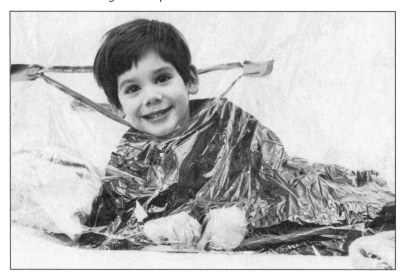

the child's arm revealed a salty taste. Instantly, the practitioner knew there was no hope of survival, and the infant died shortly thereafter.[14]

Once the characteristics and causes of CF were clearly defined, though, doctors made progress in beginning to treat different symptoms and complications effectively. For instance, Dr. Dorothy Anderson, who identified and named cystic fibrosis back in 1938, later did research that led her to recommend treating affected children with a high-calorie, high-protein, low-fat diet and with enzyme supplements she obtained from animal pancreases. The enzymes proved to be very effective in allowing normal digestion and absorption of food, and doctors still prescribe them.

Other researchers and physicians worked on developing methods of clearing out or thinning the thick mucus in CF patients' lungs. Early attempts had patients sleeping in a mist tent each night to try to thin the mucus, but this technique did not work. Some doctors prescribed a medication called acetylcysteine, since mucus in laboratory test tubes flowed more readily when this drug was added, but unfortunately human patients who inhaled it experienced irritated bronchi and breathing difficulties.

Gradually, experts developed a combination of reliable methods of clearing respiratory mucus, and today such treatments, along with the digestive aids, are the primary reason that people with CF are living longer, healthier lives.

Evaluating Individual Treatment Needs

The precise treatment regimen for a particular person depends on which organs are affected and on how severe the symptoms are. Doctors assess the types of treatment needed for the lungs by listening through a stethoscope and analyzing the results of several tests, including X rays, lung function tests, and chest scans.

X rays are usually done yearly. These images provide the physician with information on whether the lung shape has become abnormal or has deteriorated since the previous X ray. X rays also reveal whether trapped air is causing parts of the lung to swell. Lung function tests involve the patient inhaling and then exhaling into a machine called a spirometer. This machine records the amount of air exhaled. It enables doctors to detect tightening of the airways that makes breathing difficult. Chest scans are done less frequently than are X rays and lung function tests, but they are especially useful for assessing whether certain treatments, including experimental drugs, are actually effective in clearing mucus and infection. In a chest scan, the patient inhales radioactive particles that travel into the air spaces in the lungs. The particles show up under a special scanning machine, enabling a physician to see if any parts of the lungs are not receiving enough air. Sometimes the radioactive particles are injected into the bloodstream. Then, the doctor will use a scanner to monitor the blood supply to the lungs. If certain areas of the lungs appear to have insufficient air or a diminished blood supply, the doctor will prescribe more aggressive therapy.

Doctors assess the need for pancreatic enzymes by looking at the person's ability to gain weight and for symptoms of malnutrition. Sometimes they run laboratory tests on the patient's stools to analyze the chemicals and, rarely, a doctor will consider it necessary to run a tube through the nose, down the esophagus, and into the pancreas to withdraw samples of enzymes for evaluation. Usually, however, these laboratory tests are not needed because the symptoms of enzyme deficiency are obvious.

Beginning Treatment

Once a physician evaluates a CF patient to see what treatments are required, the treatment regimen will begin. Most people need some sort of daily lung and pancreas therapy in order to stay alive and grow properly.

CF treatment is usually prescribed by a family doctor, a specialist in lung or digestive disorders, or a team of health care professionals at a special cystic fibrosis clinic. Many people who do not live near such a clinic elect to travel to one of many

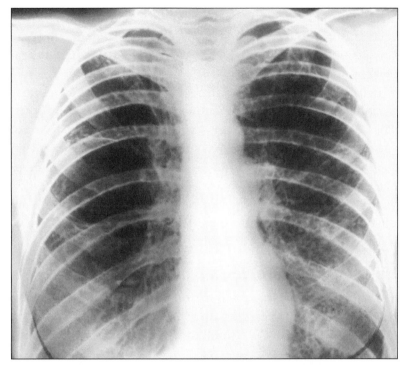

Yearly chest X rays help physicians determine the treatment necessary for CF patients.

throughout the country to at least get started on a carefully designed treatment plan. Then, a family doctor can generally monitor the patient on a regular basis, and the family can bring the person back to the CF clinic for occasional checkups or for special visits to change the therapy if complications develop.

Once experts get a CF baby or child started on a regimen, it is up to the family to administer the treatments each day. Older patients assume responsibility for their own routine care. Sometimes a patient must go to a hospital for treatment of a serious infection or other emergency, but primarily the day-to-day care is performed at home.

The goal of day-to-day care is to control symptoms as much as possible to enable the person to lead a relatively normal life. This means that the treatments must be given every day, even if the individual feels fine.

For most patients, both medicine and physical therapy are needed. Most take a dozen or more pills a day, along with some sort of inhaled medication, and schedule a half-hour physical therapy session twice a day to keep the lungs clear. As Norma, who has had CF for forty years, explains, juggling all the medications and other treatment requirements can be a major hassle. "You have to keep an eye on your many pill bottles, to make sure you don't run out. You have to plan when going on a trip, so that you have plenty for the whole time. You have to remember to take each medication at the right time, and stop it when you need to. You have to remember which ones you take to tell the doctor each time what you are taking at that time. You have to watch for med interactions and side effects."[15]

How Are Lung Problems Treated?

The primary purpose of lung treatments is to keep the airways free of mucus. Several methods can be used to achieve this goal; all are known as chest physiotherapy (CPT). Explains CF expert Dr. David M. Orenstein,

A physiotherapist helps a child and his mother perform exercises designed to rid his lungs of excess mucus.

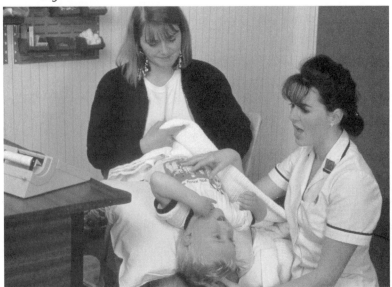

The most common method is based on a principle taken from everyday life, namely, the "Ketchup Bottle Principle." If you want to get a thick substance out of a container with a narrow opening, you turn the container upside down so that its opening is pointing downward, and then you clap it, shake it, and vibrate it. If the thick substance is mucous, and the container is the various segments of the lungs, the procedure is the same, and may be equally effective: you turn the child (or yourself) in various positions, with each position allowing one of the major portions of the lungs to have its opening pointing downward, and then you clap firmly on the back or chest over that part of the lung, and actually shake the mucous loose.[16]

Once loosened, the mucus can be coughed out.

Many people with CF use special inclined tables called postural drainage tables that slant in different ways so as to allow different parts of the lungs to drain for several minutes. The clapping on the chest or back can be performed by a family member or other caretaker using the hands or with a specialized percussion device. When this physical therapy is administered with the hands, the individual doing the procedure thumps or claps vigorously over the particular area of the lungs being drained. A patient who uses special percussion equipment has several choices. These devices do not require assistance from another person, so many teens and adults with CF prefer them to the hand techniques; however, they are very expensive, so not everyone has access to them.

One type of device is a mechanical percussor, which resembles an electric jigsaw. It has a cushion rather than a blade, and the person holds the cushion on the chest or back, where it bounces and pounds repeatedly and frees up mucus. A commercial product, the Thairapy Vest, works on a similar principle, but is worn by the patient and hooked up to a high-pressure air hose that inflates and deflates the vest, creating vibrations that loosen mucus. Also available is a percussor pack, worn like a backpack and containing a battery-operated mechanism that pounds on the back to do its job.

Several alternative methods of keeping the airways clear include the patented Flutter Valve, a small handheld device that requires the patient to blow into a tube. Inside the tube, a stainless steel ball flutters around, sending into the lungs vibrations that detach mucus from the bronchial tubes. Some people with CF say the Flutter Valve does a better job than mechanical clapping techniques, while others prefer the latter.

Another device that some patients use is the positive expiratory pressure (PEP) mask. To use this, the patient puts the mask on the face and breathes through it. This activates an exhale valve that transmits air pressure down into the airways and helps free up mucus.

Some people use a machine called a nebulizer or an aerosol inhaler to deliver mucus-breaking medication to the lungs. A drug called DNAase or Pulmozyne is most commonly employed in conjunction with CPT techniques. DNAase does not help everyone with CF, however, and it is extremely expensive—about twelve thousand dollars per year—so it is not used by the majority of CF patients.

In addition to the mucus-clearing techniques, many people with CF do special breathing exercises known as huffing. These consist of rapid, forced exhalations of air that bring up the loosened mucus so it can be coughed out. Huffing can also tell the patient whether the airways are actually getting cleared out, since a rattling sound occurs when a lot of mucus is present. When performed in conjunction with other airway clearance regimens, huffing seems to maximize the benefits and help prevent the dreaded lung infections that affect so many patients and may lead to fatal complications.

What Happens When Mucus Isn't Cleared Away?

Studies have shown that people who skip their mucus-clearing treatments are much more likely to experience deterioration in lung function, so doctors stress the importance of performing this therapy each and every day. Generally the first treatment is done in the morning to clear out mucus that has accumulated overnight. The second is done in the afternoon or evening.

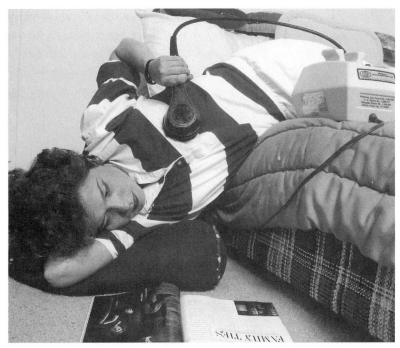

A woman uses a mechanical percussor to clear her lungs. Such a device allows CF patients more independence in treating their disease.

Although the treatments are not painful, they may come to be seen as boring intrusions on a child's playtime or on an adult's busy schedule. Small children tend to put up with the regular treatments more readily if they are allowed to play with a physioball while the parent does the CPT. This toy is about three feet around; it is specially made so the child can roll around on it during the therapy. Most teens and adults manage to get used to working the CPT into their daily schedule, and maturity brings the realization that the treatments are in large part keeping them alive.

Sometimes, despite consistent CPT treatments, trapped mucus causes breathing problems or lung infections. In such instances, many patients need to use a bronchodilator inhaler to dilate the airways so it is possible to breathe. The drugs dispensed through the inhaler are the same ones typically employed to treat asthma—albuterol, metaproterenol, or theophylline.

Patients with excessive inflammation in the airways may also need anti-inflammatory drugs like prednisone. These medications cannot be used for long periods of time because they depress the entire immune system, so doctors try to use other anti-inflammatory drugs like aspirin or ibuprofen when possible.

Antibiotic Therapies for Lung Infections

When the lungs become infected, antibiotics are used to treat the infection. These can be administered orally, through an inhaler, or intravenously in the hospital if the infection is particularly serious. Since frequent lung infections can lead to permanent scars

To treat her lung infection a girl uses an inhaler containing antibiotics.

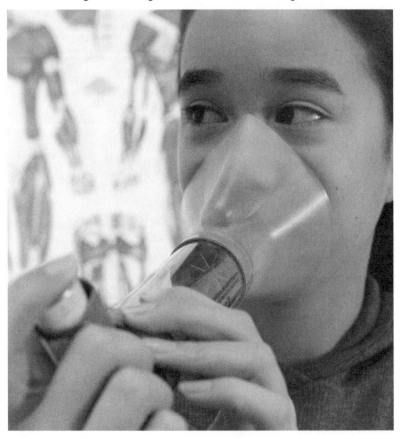

and damage, experts say it is important to clear up these infections as quickly as possible. "Controlling the episodes of increased infection and inflammation in the bronchi is the most important part of the treatment of someone with CF. The more lung damage can be prevented or delayed in someone with CF, the better and longer that person's life is likely to be,"[17] explain doctors who specialize in treating the disease.

Physicians decide on which antibiotic to use by taking a culture of the patient's sputum—the mucus coughed up from the lungs. Examining such a culture in a laboratory reveals which bacteria are present and therefore which antibiotic is likely to be most effective.

While many of the *Staphylococcus* infections frequently seen in people with CF can be treated effectively, some of the other bacteria that typically infect the lungs are resistant to drugs and less likely to respond to treatment. Two of the most troublesome resistant bacteria are *Burkholderia cepacia* and *Pseudomonas aeruginosa*. These bacteria can easily be contagious to anyone with cystic fibrosis, and for this reason many patients stay away from others in treatment for CF. This precaution may sound extreme, but many people with CF harbor these bugs throughout their lives and cannot get rid of them.

Some doctors who treat CF prescribe antibiotics to patients who do not show signs of infection, in the hope of preventing infections from getting started. However, studies have shown that this preemptive use of antibiotics helps bacteria become resistant to the very drugs that are designed to kill them. Today, most doctors do not administer antibiotics unless there are signs of an active infection.

Yet if lung infections that gain a foothold are not treated successfully, life-threatening complications can result when the progressive lung damage reaches a certain point, and this calls for immediate treatment in a hospital. The complications may include hemoptysis, in which the infection causes the person to cough up blood; atelectasis, in which a bronchial tube becomes completely blocked; pneumothorax, a collapsed lung; or complete respiratory failure. Surgery is often required for the first three complications; if the patient's condition deteriorates to respiratory failure, a mechanical ventilator may be necessary. Some people recover from respiratory failure and can gradually be weaned from the ventilator, but in most instances, this is the final complication in a long series of problems. If all other therapies fail, the patient may elect to be attached to a ventilator in an intensive care unit until death occurs.

Lung Transplants

Several years ago, there was nothing to be done for CF patients who had experienced respiratory failure. Today, though, sometimes the lives of critically ill patients can be saved with a lung transplant.

A physician will generally refer a patient to a lung transplant center when the individual develops complications that are likely to lead to death within two to three years. Many such patients require constant inhaled oxygen to survive. At the transplant center, experts evaluate the potential recipient's lungs, heart, kidneys, and other organs to determine whether the person is likely to survive a lung transplant. If the doctors believe the individual has a good chance of surviving, the person's name is placed on a transplant list until a suitable set of donor lungs becomes available. Suitability is determined by blood type, lung and body size, and how long the person has been on the list; these criteria may vary from state to state in the United States. Once the patient is near the top of the list, he or she must continually be ready to arrive at the transplant center within a few hours of receiving a call informing them that a set of lungs has become available.

Sometimes one live donor can donate a piece of one lung and a second live donor can donate a piece of the other lung, but this means that three people must have major surgery. The two live donors must also be much bigger than the recipient, since the transplanted lung pieces must fill the recipient's chest cavity. It is also difficult for surgeons to hook up the lung pieces; for these reasons experts prefer dealing with a transplant from an accident victim or other brain-dead donor if one is available. It is essential that the lungs be removed from the donor before they cease to function.

After a transplant, the recipient must remain in the hospital for several weeks or even months, until doctors are certain the new lungs are working properly and the effects of the surgical trauma have become manageable. The person must take immunosuppressive drugs for the rest of his or her life to prevent the immune system from rejecting the transplanted organ. These drugs increase susceptibility to infections and may cause diabetes, kidney problems, or other adverse effects.

The average survival rate for a CF patient who receives a lung transplant is 70 percent after one year and 48 percent after five years, so the risks associated with the procedure are high. Plus, even though a transplant gives the person a set of healthy lungs, it does not cure CF, and the digestive, reproductive, and other problems associated with the disease still remain. But many people who survive the procedure report that the risks and problems are well worth it. For the first time, many are able to do things they had only dreamed of. Darrell, for example, was so ill that he needed a lung, heart, and liver transplant at age nineteen. Prior to the operation, he was bedridden, on oxygen at all times. Afterward, he was able to participate in sports and to make college and career plans. To him, the antirejection drugs and other unpleasant things that go along with a transplant were a small price to pay for the opportunity to live a more productive life.

Experts say that people like Darrell who have a positive attitude and are willing to carefully follow their doctors' orders for ongoing posttransplant treatment are most likely to do well after such a procedure. "The patients who do the best after the operation are usually highly motivated and have a strong social-support system of family and friends,"[18] says Karen Hopkin.

Treating Digestive Problems

Treatment for the digestive problems associated with CF tends to be less complicated than that associated with the lungs, though it too must be done every day, several times per day to prevent malnutrition. Eighty-five to ninety percent of people with the disease must take pancreatic enzymes each time they eat so they can properly digest and absorb nutrients. These enzymes can be

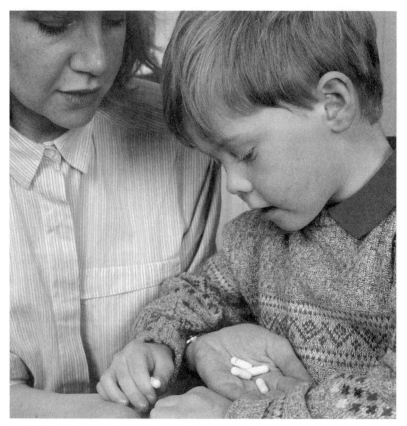

A dietician displays pills containing the pancreatic enzymes a young patient must take in order to digest his food properly.

given in powder, granule, or pill form. They are coated with a substance that prevents them from being broken down by stomach acid, so they proceed undigested to the small intestine, where the coating finally dissolves and the enzymes complete the digestion of food. Many patients take as many as twenty enzyme pills with each meal.

In addition to the pancreatic enzymes, vitamin and mineral supplements may be needed because many people with CF have trouble absorbing these essential nutrients from their food. In cases where the pancreas does not produce enough acid-neutralizing chemicals, antacids must also be taken along with these other supplements.

Usually, the correct combination of enzymes, dietary supplements, and a well-balanced, high-calorie diet is sufficient to prevent malnutrition and to allow the patient to grow in a satisfactory manner. Sometimes, though, a person with CF is still unable to gain weight and requires supplemental feedings through a tube from the nose to the stomach or through a tube directly inserted into the stomach. Patients who need feeding tubes say they are inconvenient and unpleasant, but can be tolerated, though perhaps with difficulty, by those who cannot get adequate nutrition otherwise.

The Cost of CF Treatment

All these digestive enzymes and lung-clearing medications and physical therapy devices cost a great deal of money. Often, medical insurance does not cover many of the costs, and financial concerns become an intricate part of the daily treatment regimen. Deborah, who has a son with CF, says, "Right now his meds are $2,500 a month. That doesn't include when he gets sick or hospitals or clinic visits."[19]

Some people are able to buy supplemental insurance policies to help cover costs, and some are eligible for government assistance plans like Medicaid, programs administered by Children with Special Health Needs, or Social Security. Sometimes pharmaceutical companies donate medicines to patients whose insurance will not cover these expenses. But most people affected by CF must put out large sums of money each month to pay for expensive treatments, and this adds to the already overwhelming burden of making sure that the person with cystic fibrosis receives the daily therapy he or she needs.

Chapter 4

Living with Cystic Fibrosis

A LTHOUGH IMPROVED TREATMENTS have significantly length-ened the life span for many people with cystic fibrosis, the disease is still chronic and fatal. Dealing with daily treatments, complications, and the knowledge that CF will shorten the affected person's life makes living with the disorder physically and emotionally challenging for patients and their families.

Since most patients experience health problems from birth onward and are diagnosed during early childhood, parents are initially hit hardest by the lifestyle changes and emotional impact of the disease. "When your child is diagnosed, your whole world just collapses,"[20] says Abby, who has a daughter with CF.

Common reactions to the diagnosis are terror, concern, anger, resentment, and even guilt about passing a genetic disease to a child. Some people are so distressed by the diagnosis that they deny anything is wrong. This can be very dangerous if it means that treatment is withheld as part of the denial process. Others cannot accept the reality of what is happening and challenge doctors to come up with an alternative diagnosis. Major depression is not an unusual reaction either. Many families need counseling and even antidepression medication for a while or even on an ongoing basis.

Many parents and patients who are old enough to under-stand what is happening find themselves vacillating between despair and optimism, feeling one day that they cannot deal with such a serious illness and the next day that there is good reason to believe that a cure will be found in the future.

While experts say most people are upset by a diagnosis of CF, some patients, like Shannan, actually find the diagnosis a relief. After spending the first twenty-two years of her life being misdiagnosed and therefore receiving no treatment, finding out what was actually wrong was a positive step. "My life got better once I really knew what was wrong with me. Not only were my symptoms reduced, but I also experienced a certain peace of mind in finally knowing the cause of all the health problems I had been experiencing,"[21] she said.

Shannan's experience, though, is an exception to the typical trauma that goes along with the diagnosis. Most families are particularly affected by the anxiety that comes with the realization that CF is an incurable disease with an unpredictable course of progression. "No one can predict the exact effect of cystic fibrosis on a child's lung function, growth, activity, or life span. The uncertainty is very frustrating and frightening, for it means that the family must live with the unknown from day to day,"[22] explains David Orenstein.

Methods of Easing the Trauma

Even though it is impossible to predict how CF will affect an individual, medical experts and families who deal with the disease on a daily basis say it is important to learn to accept the disorder and to work through the uncertainty and emotional upheaval. Parents especially are advised that the sooner they learn to cope, the better, since their child with CF depends on them for emotional and physical support.

Most people find that talking with family, friends, experienced health care professionals, and others who live with CF helps immensely with learning to cope with the diagnosis. Doctors, nurses, and mental health therapists affiliated with specialized CF clinics have special training in helping families adjust, but many affected persons say a compassionate and knowledgeable family doctor can be just as comforting. Contacting one of the many Internet or local, state, and national CF support groups is also immensely beneficial. Says Lenora, who has a child with CF, "The only people who really understand are other parents and individuals with CF, like those I have found on lists like Cystic-L. That support is really helpful."[23]

Families who come to accept the challenge of dealing with a chronic disease are especially well equipped to offer meaningful advice and inspiration to newly diagnosed individuals. One mother who completely revised her priorities and attitude soon after her child's diagnosis with CF, for instance, shared the following observation with other parents: "I used to wonder how anyone with a child with a terminal illness could possibly live with that knowledge. After our child was diagnosed, a light came on. We realized that life is a terminal illness and that the only time we really have is now. We just live from day to day, expecting good things."[24]

Once a parent accepts the need to make the necessary emotional and lifestyle adjustments that go along with CF, this makes it feasible to help a child learn to live with the disease as successfully as possible. Cyndi, who has had cystic fibrosis since

To measure lung function a young girl exhales into a Wright peak flow meter. Parents of CF youths are encouraged to help their children live as normally as possible.

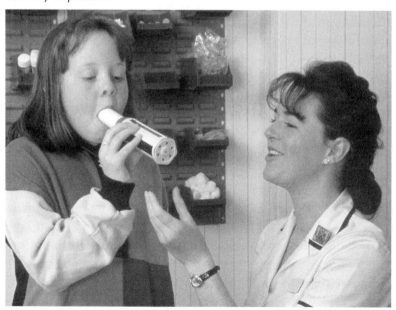

1952, tells parents that they can exert a great deal of influence over how a child with CF copes and lives day to day: "Parents have an option. They can teach their child to be well, or they can teach their child to be sick."[25]

Experts say that a major component in teaching a child to be well is explaining things in a positive, yet honest manner. Telling a child who is old enough to understand that they will feel better if they take their medicine and receive CPT treatments each day is an example of how a parent might incorporate a positive attitude into a discussion of CF. Researching the disease thoroughly and thus being able to answer questions calmly and accurately is also recommended as a good way of helping the child cope and develop a positive outlook.

Doctors who specialize in treating CF also advise parents not to baby or overprotect the young patient. This means allowing the child to participate in normal childhood activities as much as the individual's physical condition permits. "Children with CF should be treated normally: they need to do homework and chores, and should be allowed to participate in all normal childhood activities. Children treated this way grow up healthier emotionally and physically,"[26] says David Orenstein. Jenny, an adult who has CF, credits the fact that her parents treated her just like they treated her three siblings, who do not have CF, with helping her lead a normal, productive childhood and with teaching her to accept responsibility for her own care. Jenny believes that her mom and dad's attitude also taught her to push herself to achieve her goals despite medical obstacles that stood in the way.

Day-to-Day Adjustments

No matter how successfully patients and families cope with the impact of CF, many lifestyle adjustments must be made to accommodate daily treatments and rise to meet medical emergencies. Once these adjustments are in place, however, things can change at a moment's notice, calling for new adjustments. A child who goes to school and participates in sports, for example, may suddenly develop a lung infection and have to be isolated from schoolmates and others for a lengthy stretch of time. Conversely, someone who was too sick to go to school may receive a new medication that results in marked improvement, enabling him or her to start school for the first time.

According to affected persons, one of the biggest parts of adjusting to life with CF is getting accustomed to spending a great deal of time with doctor visits and daily treatments. Some people consult a primary care physician and specialists to deal with lung, digestive, or reproductive matters as needed, while others go to a specialized CF center that may be some distance away.

Studies show that patients who go to specialized clinics have higher survival rates, but traveling to such a facility imposes practical burdens. These visits disrupt work and school schedules, leisure activities, and household chores. Children in the family who do not have CF may require other care arrangements and may feel neglected. Marriages may become strained because of emotional, physical, and financial issues.

Growing Up with CF

Getting used to the daily treatments may also be difficult for the patient and family. Some children resent having to take medication and do not like sitting still for chest physiotherapy sessions, and some are embarrassed about having to take enzyme pills at school before eating. Some children are teased by their peers because of the pills or because they cough, but most families find that if a parent or teacher takes the time to explain what is going on to classmates, the taunting goes away. Usually a child with CF who maintains a positive, matter-of-fact attitude manages to convince others that CF treatments are a necessary but not insurmountable part of daily life. Seven-year-old Billy, for example, gets his medications and breathing treatments at home before leaving for school. Then, at lunchtime he takes his pancreatic enzymes in the nurse's office and eats lunch with his classmates. After school, he gets more breathing treatments at home, often with his friends present. But since Billy accepts the need to take a half hour out of playtime to get the treatments, his friends accept it, too. According to his mom,

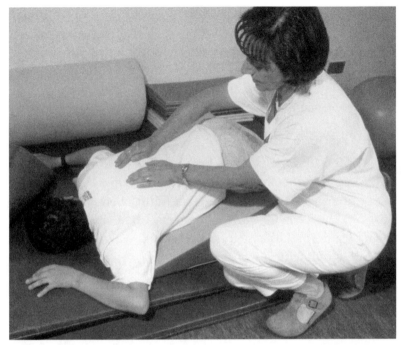

A young man receives percussion treatment from a physiotherapist. Young people often find it difficult to fit CF therapies into their hectic schedules.

Daelynn, Billy's attitude has set the tone for a healthy, normal-as-possible childhood, and in addition has taught those around him what is really important and relevant in life. "He has especially taught me not to sweat the small stuff, there's more important things than if he wears the same shirt for 2 months (his latest quest is to wear the same shirt all school year) or doesn't like to wear underwear. Those are small things in the bigger picture of our lives."[27]

Young people who are older than Billy, especially teenagers, may have a more difficult time accepting and dealing with daily treatments because of the normal questioning and rebellion that come with the teen years. The opinion of peers is especially important to teens, and having CF can introduce a nightmare into the quest for acceptance, according to some patients. Many teens with CF experience delayed sexual maturation, too, which can make fitting in even more difficult.

Some teens with CF reportedly go through a very difficult phase in which they resist keeping up their treatments, and sometimes this requires counseling and other professional intervention. Experts say that in most instances, though, a teen who previously accepted the need for daily treatment will manage to continue the program.

Every Aspect of Life

Besides the lifestyle changes that directly involve daily treatments, people affected by CF say it has an impact on virtually every other aspect of a family's daily life. Lenora, whose six-year-old child has CF, for example, says that she is rarely able to enjoy a normal lunch hour at work because she is constantly battling with medical insurance matters:

> The insurance thing absolutely sucks, no matter how great a company you are dealing with. It seems there is always a misunderstanding or a bill that shouldn't be coming to us or something that isn't covered. You have to call over and over and listen to the company message while on hold for what seems

A child uses an inhaler at school; this device is also used by CF patients.

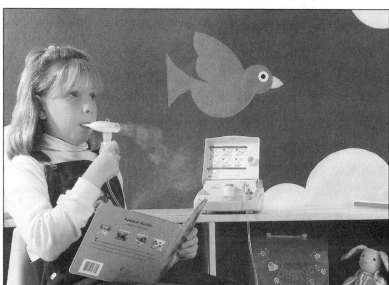

like hours at a time. It all sounds trivial, but it just reinforces all the time that we are different. Most other parents are not spending their lunch hours on hold for an insurance company.[28]

Other aspects of life that most people are not bothered by also become central issues when CF is concerned. One example is the importance of keeping someone with CF away from cigarette smoke. While recent studies have shown that secondhand smoke is harmful to everyone, it is imperative that people with cystic fibrosis avoid it to prevent lung complications. This means that no one in the person's home may smoke, and if the patient visits someone else's home or even a restaurant or other public place, it is essential that they not be around anyone who is smoking. This can create awkward situations; for instance, what if a child with CF is playing in a park and someone nearby lights a cigarette?

Affected families say other seemingly routine ventures can also take on gargantuan proportions. Something as simple as planning a family vacation can become a complicated ordeal. An ordinary camping trip is out of the question, as Linda, who has a son with CF, reveals:

> After our son was dxed [diagnosed] at six months we made the decision to purchase a small twenty-four-foot motor home so we could continue with our vacations. We love to camp, but there is no way that Travis can handle the heat; he needs AC, has meds that have to be refrigerated, and needs electricity for nebs [nebulizers] and [the percussor] vest. We spent our "nest egg" on the RV so that we could enjoy our family vacations now. So far Travis has been very healthy, and we want to take advantage of that because no one knows what the future holds.[29]

Making the Best of Each Day

Despite the impact of accommodating CF in endeavors like vacations and trips to the park, like Travis's family, many people who live with CF today are able to maintain a positive attitude and to live reasonably full, though not normal, lives, doing things that would not have been possible thirty years ago. Different patients and family members attribute their ability to forge ahead and do their best to different forces and techniques, but most share a powerful drive to succeed despite all odds and a sense of contagious optimism about recent progress in treatment and the hope of an eventual cure.

Actress Kathi Novelli, for instance, who was diagnosed with CF when she was six months old, says, "I never give up hope. I always follow my dream. If I stopped doing theater, if I stopped my normal routine, I know my health would get the better of me."[30]

Marathon runner and physician Ken Subin, who lost a brother to CF, also pushed himself to achieve incredible goals despite having cystic fibrosis: "After witnessing the devastating effects of CF firsthand, I was determined to beat the odds. I knew that to do that, I would have to put my physical health above all else and do everything within my power to stay healthy. For me, this included getting adequate sleep, exercising and maintaining proper nutrition."[31] In addition to becoming a physician, Subin completed his first marathon at age thirty-one.

For some people with CF, the motivation and drive to go on derive from actively participating in clinical trials and social activities related to the disease. Eric, for example, who has had CF for over thirty years, regularly signs up for clinical trials that can help himself and others with CF. He has also testified before a U.S. Senate subcommittee on public health to stress the importance of gene therapy research. Beth, a lawyer who has CF, volunteers to help other patients with legal and insurance matters, including special school accommodations and job discrimination issues. Myra, a mom who has two children with CF, volunteers tirelessly for CF-related causes and has helped raise over $1 million in research funds.

Still Some Limitations

Despite all the positive stories of patients and families living successfully with cystic fibrosis, many avenues still remain closed to people with the disease. While many careers are open to those who wish to pursue them, most people with CF cannot choose careers that would expose them to smoke, dust, or chemical

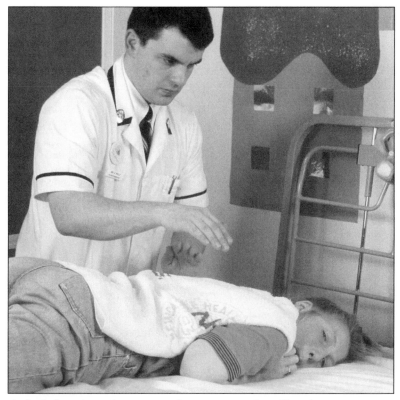

A physiotherapist performs percussion on a young boy. Though many avenues are open to those with CF, a career in medicine is usually not advised.

fumes. Experts say it is also not a good idea for most people with CF to enter the teaching or medical professions, where they would frequently be exposed to cold viruses and other respiratory infections.

Laws such as the Americans with Disabilities Act prohibit employers from discriminating against anyone with a disease like CF. Nonetheless, people with the disorder are often denied employment or promotions. While it is possible to pursue legal action in such instances, this can be costly and time consuming. Many individuals who do not have the necessary funds or time allotment are not able to do anything about such instances of discrimination and experience professional setbacks and other hardships due to these kinds of events.

Another area that remains outside the normal range of opportunities for people with CF is bearing children. Most men with CF are infertile, which means that fatherhood is impossible for these individuals. Some women with the disease are able to conceive, but carrying a baby to term would most likely be detrimental to the patient's lung function. The risks of stillbirth or premature birth are also higher for a woman with CF, and the fact that a baby can inherit the disease is also a consideration. The knowledge that a parent with CF is not likely to live long enough to see a child reach adulthood is another factor that keeps most patients from reproducing.

Experts say that as medical science continues to prolong the lives of people with CF, childbearing will become an option for more and more affected persons. Now that it is possible for doctors to assess whether a developing fetus will be born with CF, families are able to receive prenatal testing to determine whether abnormal CF genes are present. The eventual development of methods of correcting the underlying causes of CF will remove one more barrier for those with CF who wish to reproduce.

The End of Life with CF

With all the modern progress that has allowed so many people with CF to lead increasingly normal and fulfilling lives, the disease still shortens their life span, and the prospect of death still rears its unwelcome head when things take a turn for the worse. This adds significant sadness and stress to the patient and family's lives, particularly if the patient is a child, but since most people with CF die from the disease rather than from old age, it is an event for which all must prepare.

Most individuals with CF succumb to respiratory failure when the lungs can no longer provide oxygen and remove carbon dioxide from the body. This generally results from a gradual process of deterioration, and during the ordeal, many decisions about relieving the patient's discomfort and placing him or her in a hospital or hospice facility must be made. The comfort and counseling that many hospices provide lead many families to agree that a loved one's last days should be spent in such an environment, but some choose to remain at home or to enter a regular hospital where maximum life support and pain relief are available.

The end, of course, is never easy, and the impact of losing a loved one drives some individuals to unrelenting despair and mourning. But many people, even parents of children who succumb to CF, learn to find a measure of peace by emphasizing the blessings that the person brought into their lives. Writes one mother,

> Sarah was in our lives for 10 3/4 years and taught us a lot. We learnt the value of simple things in life, like being together and loving each other. We learnt to pull together in difficult times and not shut each other out. We learnt that no person is an island and how much we need each other. We learnt how much we love our children and how we must never take them for granted. We are grateful to God for giving us such a wonderful, special child.[32]

Chapter 5

The Future

D ESPITE THE FACT that improved treatments have increased the quality and duration of life for many people with cystic fibrosis, the disease still causes incalculable suffering and premature death, and patients, their families, and medical experts look forward to the day when CF will be curable. Scientists now know what is necessary to achieve such a cure, and the challenge for the future is to develop the techniques necessary for bridging the gap between theoretical knowledge and a workable solution.

Experts say that a cure for CF would require fixing the defect that prevents the chloride channels controlled by CFTR from working properly. Investigators are focusing on three main areas of research to achieve this goal: gene therapy, protein repair and chloride channel activation, and drug therapy. "The cure," according to experts at the Cystic Fibrosis Foundation, "most likely will combine all three."[33]

Gene Therapy

Ever since 1989, when researchers identified the defective CFTR genes as the underlying cause of cystic fibrosis, experts have been optimistic about developing a method of replacing faulty genes with normal ones to cure the disease. This avenue of research is known as gene therapy; unfortunately it has proven to be much more difficult than originally anticipated to actually achieve the desired results.

In 1990 several teams of scientists figured out how to make a normal CFTR gene and used it to correct the abnormal CFTR protein product in test tubes and animal models in a laboratory setting. At that time, many people thought a cure for CF was close at hand. But when doctors tried to introduce the normal gene into the lungs or nasal passages of human patients starting in 1993, the results were not as encouraging. In order to insert the gene into the respiratory system, the investigators needed a DNA-containing substance called a vector. They chose a modified adenovirus (a virus that causes the common cold), but this approach turned out to be unreliable.

Doctors administered the virus and gene with nose drops or through a flexible tube leading into a patient's lungs. They reasoned that since the adenovirus normally infects these areas, it should go right for the cells with the defective CFTR genes that

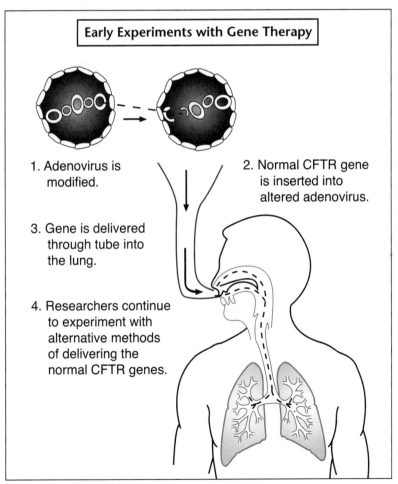

Early Experiments with Gene Therapy

1. Adenovirus is modified.

2. Normal CFTR gene is inserted into altered adenovirus.

3. Gene is delivered through tube into the lung.

4. Researchers continue to experiment with alternative methods of delivering the normal CFTR genes.

needed replacing. But even though the modified adenovirus had been genetically altered so as not to actually cause an infection in the people undergoing treatment, the patient's immune systems still detected the virus as an invader and launched an immune attack. This prevented the normal genes from replacing the defective ones. The virus and normal genes also did not stay in the patient's body long enough to make a difference, which was another problem that researchers realized had to be solved. It would be necessary to not only find a reliable method of delivering the normal genes to the lung epithelial cells, but also develop a way of prolonging the genes' residence time in the cells.

To surmount the immune system and durability problems, researchers started working on alternative methods of delivering the normal gene. In 1995 scientists at the University of Alabama at Birmingham began testing a way of delivering healthy CFTR genes with fat capsules known as liposomes. Another group at Johns Hopkins University Hospital started testing a different viral vector called an adeno-associated virus. This is a type of animal virus that does not normally infect humans, so is less likely to trigger an immune response, but is very likely to get into the recipient's cellular DNA where it is needed. That same year, a third group of researchers at Massachusetts General Hospital in Boston began experimenting with an aerosol version of the adenovirus–normal gene vector to see if that would help solve the delivery problem.

New Approaches in a New Century

Early results with these alternative methods of delivery proved to be no more reliable than those with the original adenovirus, and thus far the search for an effective vector system that manages to avoid an immune system attack while being durable enough to remain in the appropriate cells is continuing. Different researchers are currently experimenting with a variety of viral and nonviral vectors, including liposomes and adeno-associated viruses. One recent approach that seems promising is combining two viruses to take advantage of the individual characteristics of each. A team of investigators at the University of Pennsylvania in

Philadelphia is using a disabled form of the human immuno-deficiency virus (HIV), which causes acquired immune deficiency syndrome (AIDS), and a disabled form of the lethal Ebola virus, which causes hemorrhagic fever, to deliver healthy CFTR genes into the epithelial cells lining the lungs of people with CF. Both viruses are carefully modified so as not to cause disease, and the researchers believe the combination holds a great deal of promise because of the capacity of Ebola to penetrate lung cells and the ability of HIV to stay inside a host cell for long periods of time.

Another brand-new avenue of gene delivery research is testing a compacted DNA nanoparticle known as PLASmin for use as a vector. Nanoparticles are tiny chemical compounds whose properties change according to their size. They have a wide variety of biological and engineering applications, including getting into cells in the body in an efficient manner. Experts led by Dr. Michael Konstan, affiliated with Copernicus Therapeutics at the University Hospitals of Cleveland, Case Western Reserve University School of Medicine, and Cystic Fibrosis Foundation Therapeutics, are attempting to use PLASmin to breach lung cell membranes to deliver a normal gene directly to the cell nucleus. The compacted substance does not trigger an immune response in laboratory animals, and investigators hope it will display this characteristic in humans as well.

Besides developing reliable methods of delivering normal CFTR genes directly into the lungs of people with CF, gene therapy researchers also hope to expand their efforts to correct the faulty gene in body parts other than the lungs. Thus far most work has centered on the lungs because they are easily accessible through the nose and throat and because the lungs are the most common site of life-threatening damage associated with CF. But in the future, scientists hope to progress to the point of also targeting cells in the pancreas and other areas affected by the disorder.

Protein Repair and Chloride Channel Research

Along with efforts to develop a reliable method of replacing the faulty genes that underlie cystic fibrosis, scientists are also focusing on a related area as part of the overall drive to improve

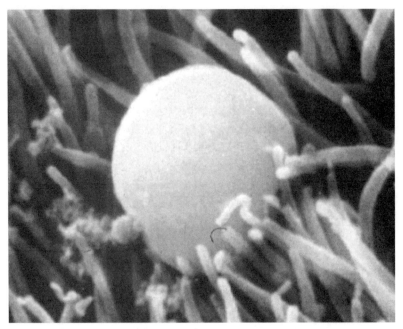

Research on protein assist therapies is currently under way so that mucous (magnified in this view) production may be eliminated.

treatments and cure the disease. With the set of techniques known as protein assist or repair therapies, investigators attempt to correct the abnormal CFTR protein in order to allow the cells of people with CF to reach a normal salt balance and therefore eliminate the sticky, thick mucus that forms. The closely related field of chloride channel therapies, rather than correcting the abnormal CFTR protein, introduces other proteins that allow the cells to properly process salt.

One example of a protein assist therapy under investigation is being conducted at the University of Alabama at Birmingham, where patients are receiving the antibiotics gentamicin or tobramycin through the nose to see if these drugs enhance the activity of CFTR protein, thus enabling the lungs to clear out mucus. Studies at several other research centers are looking at methods of activating alternative chloride channels that will result in the same end. A new drug called INS37217, which is designed to stimulate the movement of chloride and water out of cells in the lungs and nasal passages, is being tested for this purpose. Preliminary results show that this drug may be valuable in promoting airway clearance because it increases the water content of mucus, making it easier for the patient to expel the unwanted substance.

Other researchers are attempting to synthesize other chloride ion channel proteins that would allow the movement of salt across the membranes of the epithelial cells of people with CF. Dr. John Tomich of Kansas State University, for example, has put together a synthetic mini-protein that produces chloride ion channels just like whole proteins do. Tomich is currently testing a method of administering the mini-protein to CF patients. A recent article in the *Kansas State Collegian* is cautiously optimistic: "The envisioned drug therapy, developed by Tomich, would be a device similar to an inhaler that would disperse synthetic mini-proteins into the body to produce cross channels for chloride ions and fluids to pass through."[34]

Related studies are trying to find out as much as possible about all the different abnormal proteins involved in the movement of chloride ions in CF. The goal of such studies is to eventually develop ways of controlling these proteins. A joint project by Proteome Systems of Sydney, Australia, and Cystic Fibrosis Foundation Therapeutics of Bethesda, Maryland, for instance, has the intention of performing a comprehensive analysis of these proteins. Explains researcher Dr. Jenny Harry of Proteome Systems, "We are interested in identifying protein expression patterns specific to the sputum and lung secretions of CF individuals. Once these unique proteins are identified, the next step is to develop drugs to prevent the action or interactions of these proteins, thereby reducing chronic CF lung disease and delaying the need for treatments such as heart-lung transplants."[35]

Developing New Drugs

The third major area of present and future investigation, the development of new drugs, overlaps with some of the experimental protein repair therapies, and in addition seeks to target other specific problems such as infection and inflammation associated with CF.

New drugs are originally invented and tested on animals in a laboratory. Once a compound has been proven to be safe and effective in a laboratory setting, the drug developer may apply to the Food and Drug Administration (FDA) in the United States or to comparable agencies in other countries to begin testing on humans in clinical trials. Three phases are generally involved in a clinical trial. Phase 1 lasts several months and is designed to determine safe doses and methods of administration and to track any adverse effects that may occur. For example, in Phase 1 doctors determine whether the drug should be given by mouth, injected, or inhaled. Only a few patients, seldom more than twenty, participate in Phase 1 trials. All are volunteers who are informed that the drug being tested may or may not help them. People can volunteer for clinical trials through physicians participating in the study or by contacting various research centers that advertise the trials online or through cystic fibrosis support groups.

When Phase 1 trials show that a new drug appears to help people and to be without dangerous adverse effects, Phase 2 may begin. Here, more volunteer patients, perhaps as many as one hundred, are given the new drug to further establish safety and effectiveness. If carefully analyzed test results indicate that the drug is extremely safe and effective, the manufacturer may apply to the FDA for so-called fast-track testing status so the medication can be made available promptly for widespread Phase 3 testing. If, on the other hand, questions remain as to whether the drug is indeed safe and worthwhile for the purpose it was developed, it may be sent back to the laboratory for modification or simply dropped from further trials at this point.

In Phase 3, which can last several years, hundreds or even thousands of volunteers are randomly assigned to either experimental or control groups to objectively test the drug's effectiveness. Patients in a control group are unknowingly given a placebo, or fake that looks like the real thing. This control is necessary because sometimes volunteers who receive the placebo in clinical trials experience positive effects simply because they hope and expect to be helped. Thus if results from the control and experimental groups are very similar, scientists cannot rule out the possibility that expectations that the new drug will work, rather than the medication's therapeutic properties, are responsible for any perceived healing. If, on the other hand, researchers determine that a sufficient number of people in the experimental groups show marked improvement compared with those in the placebo groups, doctors can attribute the positive results to the drug itself.

Once Phase 3 is completed in a satisfactory manner, the FDA may approve the new drug for marketing. Sometimes a drug manufacturer will continue testing into Phase 4 to further study long-term safety, but this is not required.

After a drug has successfully completed clinical trials, doctors can begin prescribing the new compound for patients not enrolled in the trials. So that many patients have access to truly promising new drugs as soon as possible, many CF clinics and organizations like the Cystic Fibrosis Foundation have set up programs that constantly monitor new drug development and testing and inform doctors when these medications become available for widespread use.

New Drugs Being Tested

Since most life-threatening complications associated with CF are related to infection and inflammation in the lungs, many researchers are testing new drugs that effectively treat these problems. Investigators have discovered, for example, that much of the dangerous airway inflammation results from an accumulation of large numbers of immune system cells called neutrophils. Thus, several drugs are being studied that have the ability to block neutrophils from inflaming lung tissue. One such compound, BIIL284BS, works by blocking the response of neutrophils to chemical signals produced by an inflamed lung. Researchers have begun Phase 1 trials on cystic fibrosis patients and hope that this drug will prove to be effective in safely reducing lung inflammation.

Related research is testing interleukin 10 (IL-10), a naturally occurring protein that normally reduces inflammation. Researchers have found that people with CF tend to make abnormally low amounts of IL-10, and they are hoping that giving these patients a synthetic version of this protein will help alleviate lung inflammation.

Several investigators are looking into other new ways of protecting the lungs of people with CF from infection. One approach is using a new type of aerosol medication known as an antimicrobial peptide. Peptides are organic chemical compounds constructed of amino acids. Antimicrobial peptides have

A nurse gives an antibiotic treatment to a woman with a respiratory infection. Scientists are testing many drugs to fight the bacteria and virus responsible for such common infections.

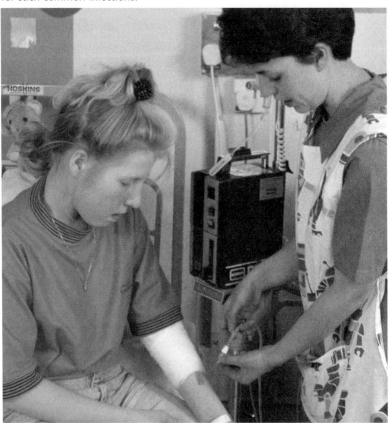

the ability to kill germs. Scientists are developing synthetic antimicrobial peptides that are similar to naturally occurring chemicals that protect the lungs from infection. One such experimental peptide, IB367, is the first of its class to be tested, and investigators are hopeful that, if it is effective, it will introduce a whole new avenue of therapy for preventing lung infections.

Other scientists are testing new antibiotics in hopes of more successfully treating the many dangerous lung infections that plague CF patients. The new antibiotic meropenum, for instance, seems to work not only against the *Pseudomonas* bacteria that commonly cause such infections, but also against *Burkholderia cepacia*, which is difficult to eradicate and tends to be resistant to most antibiotics. *Burkholderia cepacia* is, in fact, such a serious concern for patients that entire laboratories have been set up to study methods of killing it. At the Cystic Fibrosis Foundation's Burkholderia Cepacia Research Laboratory and Repository at the University of Michigan in Ann Arbor, for example, researchers are identifying different strains of the bacteria in lung secretions of CF patients to try to develop new drugs against these different strains. The investigators are also trying to develop reliable methods of deciding on the best course of therapy for individuals with specific strains.

Since scientists completed mapping the entire genome (genetic structure) of *Pseudomonas aeruginosa* in 2000, doctors have been hopeful that this accomplishment will lead to new drugs that target specific genetic components and are thus particularly effective in arresting the growth of this bacteria. Efforts are under way to map the genomes of other bacteria that affect CF patients so that these too may be targeted.

One additional new avenue of drug research is attempting to combat not a bacterial source of lung infections, but a virus called respiratory syncytial virus. This virus is responsible for many CF-associated lung infections, and scientists have recently developed artificial antibodies that fight the virus. Studies are under way to test the effectiveness of injecting these antibodies once a month as a sort of vaccine to try to prevent related lung infections.

Other Areas of Research

Besides the three main areas of cystic fibrosis research—gene therapy, protein repair, and new drugs—several additional avenues of current investigation aim to improve the quality of life for people with the disease.

Some researchers are looking at methods of improving existing therapies. For example, doctors at several research centers are comparing airway clearance techniques like the Flutter Valve, the Thairapy Vest, and standard hand percussion CPT to determine exactly what variables make different techniques best for different patients. Related research is exploring the feasibility of combining the use of aerosol medications and physical airway clearance techniques. Doctors are testing whether patients can effectively use the Thairapy Vest, which vibrates against the chest wall to free trapped mucus, while inhaling aerosol medicines that help clear the airways. Presently, many patients use both of these therapies, but separately, and researchers hope that combining them will prove to be more effective and also save a great deal of time that the person must devote to daily treatments.

An entirely different kind of research is investigating the value of different nutritional supplements in improving weight gain and overall growth in children with CF. One promising compound being tested at Johns Hopkins University Hospital contains special calcium supplements; at other centers, doctors are exploring whether other types of vitamin and mineral combinations are helpful.

Many researchers are also concerned with trying to improve methods of assessing how far the disease has progressed in certain individuals. One group of studies is investigating whether computerized tomography (CT) scans, a sophisticated technique that enables doctors to see images of various internal body parts, is an accurate method of measuring mucous plugs and lung inflammation in CF patients. Other researchers are looking at whether certain chemicals in the blood accurately reveal the extent of lung inflammation. At the present time

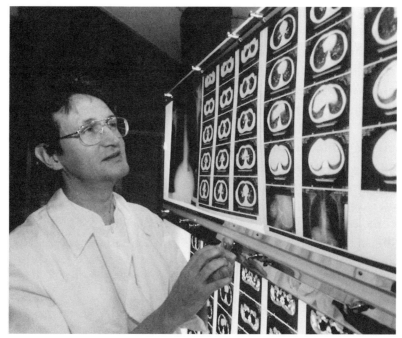

A cystic fibrosis specialist studies computerized tomography (CT) scans in hopes of measuring lung inflammation and mucous plugs more effectively in the future.

there are no blood tests that precisely measure this variable, and doctors hope that one can be developed that can give a quick, reliable assessment of how the lungs are doing at a particular time.

How Long Before There Is a Cure?

The ultimate goal of all this ongoing research is to continue to improve the quality and length of life for people with CF and to achieve a cure—an elusive goal that presently seems so close and yet so far away. As more and more patients live longer, more productive lives, there is an ever-growing sense that many children born today with CF will see a cure within their lifetime. While no one can estimate exactly when such a cure will materialize, experts and affected people alike share a healthy optimism that in this era of unprecedented technology, each day brings scientists closer and closer to this aim.

The past three decades alone have taken cystic fibrosis from being a disease that killed most children it affected before their fifth birthday to one that is increasingly a disease of adulthood as well as childhood. The Cystic Fibrosis Foundation, an organization that has helped countless patients and families with information, support, and research efforts, has chosen the motto "adding tomorrows every day" to represent the ongoing progress that surrounds the disease, and their message that "with each sunrise, scientists understand a bit more about the disease; promising new drugs advance through the pipeline; and caregivers' techniques to manage the symptoms of CF become more powerful"[36] gives hope and a sense of purpose to the many individuals who have good reason to be excited about the future.

Notes

Introduction: No Longer Just a Childhood Disease

1. Cystic Fibrosis Foundation, "Teacher's Guide," www.cff.org.
2. Quoted in Cystic Fibrosis Foundation, "The Story of 65 Roses," www.cff.org.
3. Roland Merullo, "Of Young Life and Breath," *Philadelphia Inquirer*, April 7, 2002, p. 3.

Chapter 1: What Is Cystic Fibrosis?

4. Quoted in David M. Orenstein, M.D., *Cystic Fibrosis: A Guide for Patient and Family*. Philadelphia: Lippincott-Raven, 1997, p. 343.
5. Karen Hopkin, Ph.D., *Understanding Cystic Fibrosis*. Jackson: University of Mississippi Press, 1998, p. 26.
6. Cystic Fibrosis Foundation, "Sweat Testing," www.cff.org.
7. Orenstein, *Cystic Fibrosis*, p. 17.
8. Jane Braverman, Ph.D., "Cystic Fibrosis No Longer a Fatal Disease," *The Exceptional Parent Magazine*, November 2001, p. 32.

Chapter 2: What Causes Cystic Fibrosis?

9. Howard Hughes Medical Institute, "Stalking a Lethal Gene: Finding the Faulty Gene's Fellow Travelers," 2002. www.hhmi.org.
10. Mayo Clinic.com, "What Is Cystic Fibrosis?" 2002. www.mayoclinic.com.
11. Mayo Clinic.com, "What Is Cystic Fibrosis?"
12. Hopkin, *Understanding Cystic Fibrosis*, p. 16.

13. Pulmonology Channel, "Cystic Fibrosis," 2001. www.pul monologychannel.com.

Chapter 3: Treatment

14. Zoe A. Davis, M.S., P.N.P., R.N., "Cystic Fibrosis," *Nurse week.com*, May 7, 2002. www.nurseweek.com.
15. Norma Kennedy Plourde, interview by author, September 24, 2002.
16. Orenstein, *Cystic Fibrosis*, p. 38.
17. Orenstein, *Cystic Fibrosis*, p. 34.
18. Hopkin, *Understanding Cystic Fibrosis*, p. 70.
19. Deborah Irizarry, interview by author, September 20, 2002.

Chapter 4: Living with Cystic Fibrosis

20. Quoted in Merullo, "Of Young Life and Breath," p. 1.
21. Quoted in Cystic Fibrosis Foundation, "Shannan Burk," www.cff.org.
22. Orenstein, *Cystic Fibrosis*, p. 219.
23. Lenora Degen, interview by author, September 20, 2002.
24. Hopkin, *Understanding Cystic Fibrosis*, p. 77.
25. Quoted in Braverman, "Cystic Fibrosis No Longer a Fatal Disease," p. 34.
26. Orenstein, *Cystic Fibrosis*, p. 217.
27. Daelynn Williams, interview by author, September 24, 2002.
28. Degen, interview, September 20, 2002.
29. Linda Kennedy, interview by author, September 20, 2002.
30. Quoted in Cystic Fibrosis Foundation, "Kathi Novelli," www.cff.org.
31. Quoted in Cystic Fibrosis Foundation, "Ken Subin, M.D.," www.cff.org.
32. Quoted in Hopkin, *Understanding Cystic Fibrosis*, p. 82.

Chapter 5: The Future

33. Cystic Fibrosis Foundation, "Gene Therapy and CF," www. cff.org.
34. David Lott, "K-State, KU Develop Cystic Fibrosis Treatment," *Kansas State University Collegian*, June 9, 1997. www.kstatecol legian.com.

35. Quoted in Cystic Fibrosis Foundation, "Strategic Alliance on Proteomics of CF Announced," March 18, 2002. www.cff.org.

36. Cystic Fibrosis Foundation, "Living with CF," www.cff.org.

Glossary

acini: Cells in the pancreas that manufacture digestive enzymes.

adenovirus: A virus that causes the common cold; when modified it may be used to carry a normal gene into the airways of CF patients.

aerosol: A method of administering medication via an inhaled mist.

airways: The tubes that carry air in and out of the lungs.

bronchi: Airways connecting the windpipe and the lungs.

bronchitis: An inflammation of the major airways leading to the lungs.

carrier: A person who carries a defective gene but does not develop a related disease.

CFTR: The cystic fibrosis transmembrane conductance regulator gene and the protein made by the gene responsible for CF.

chloride channel: The tiny gate through which chloride ions pass as they move through a cell membrane.

chromosome: The wormlike bodies that house genes in the cell nucleus.

cystic fibrosis: A disease characterized by thick, sticky mucus that prevents the lungs, pancreas, and other organs from functioning properly.

digestive enzymes: Chemicals that help the body digest food; many digestive enzymes are produced by the pancreas.

ducts: Passages or tubes that carry secretions from glands.

epithelial cells: Cells that line the body's exocrine glands and other organs affected by CF.

exocrine glands: Glands that secrete chemicals through ducts.

gene: The basic unit of hereditary information.

genetic marker: Certain sequences of DNA that appear in families of people with a particular disease.

huffing: Forced rapid exhalation to loosen trapped mucus in the lungs.

ion: A charged atomic particle.

mucus: Slimy fluid secreted by certain cells in organs and glands.

nebulizer: A device that converts a liquid medication into an inhaled mist.

percussion: Clapping or thumping on the chest or back to dislodge mucus from the lungs.

sputum: Mucus coughed up from the lungs.

vector: In gene therapy, the substance that carries the therapeutic gene into the patient's body.

Organizations to Contact

Cystic Fibrosis Foundation
6931 Arlington Road
Bethesda, MD 20814
(301) 951-4422
(800) 344-4823
website: www.cff.org

The primary organization for CF support and information in the United States; provides a comprehensive website covering disease description, treatment, research, personal stories, and referrals to local chapters and CF clinics.

Cystic Fibrosis Research Incorporated
Bayside Business Plaza
2672 Bayshore Parkway, Suite 520
Mountain View, CA 94043
(650) 404-9975
website: www.cfri.org

Nonprofit organization dedicated to funding CF research and providing educational and support services to patients and their families.

Cystic Fibrosis Worldwide
Bosbes 12
5708 DA Helmond/The Netherlands
+31.492.520241
website: www.cfww.org

International organization that offers news, information, and support through conferences, newsletters, and website.

For Further Reading

Books

Jane Chumbley, *Cystic Fibrosis: A Family Affair.* London: Sheldon Press, 1999. Special section for young adults with CF; information on research, treatment, and coping for the whole family.

Ann Harris, *Cystic Fibrosis: The Facts.* Oxford, UK: Oxford University Press, 1995. Easily understood, comprehensive book on cystic fibrosis.

Andy Lipman, *Alive at 25: How I'm Beating Cystic Fibrosis.* Marietta, GA: Longstreet Press, 2001. An inspirational account of a young man's struggles and triumphs over cystic fibrosis.

Websites

CF Web Home Page (www.ai.mit.edu). An index of appropriate Internet sites and support services.

Cystic Fibrosis Mutation Database (www.genet.sickkids.on.ca). Provides information on many of the gene mutations that cause CF.

Cystic-L (www.cystic-l.org). A free e-mail service that offers information and support for people with CF.

Works Consulted

Books

Karen Hopkin, Ph.D., *Understanding Cystic Fibrosis.* Jackson: University Press of Mississippi, 1998. Comprehensive information, written in an easily understood manner, on the disease, causes, treatment, research, and living with CF.

David M. Orenstein, M.D., *Cystic Fibrosis: A Guide for Patient and Family.* Philadelphia: Lippincott-Raven, 1997. Very well-written, comprehensive book about the disease by one of the world's foremost CF experts.

Periodicals

Jane Braverman, Ph.D., "Cystic Fibrosis No Longer a Fatal Disease," *The Exceptional Parent Magazine*, November 2001.

Roland Merullo, "Of Young Life and Breath," *Philadelphia Inquirer*, April 7, 2002.

Michael J. Welsh and Alan E. Smith, "Cystic Fibrosis," *Scientific American*, December 1995.

Internet Sources

Cystic Fibrosis Foundation, "Gene Therapy and CF," www.cff.org.

Cystic Fibrosis Foundation, "Kathi Novelli," www.cff.org.

Cystic Fibrosis Foundation, "Ken Subin, M.D.," www.cff.org.

Cystic Fibrosis Foundation, "Living with CF," www.cff.org.

Cystic Fibrosis Foundation, "Shannan Burk," www.cff.org.

Cystic Fibrosis Foundation, "The Story of 65 Roses," www.cff.org.

Cystic Fibrosis Foundation, "Strategic Alliance on Proteomics of CF Announced," March 18, 2002. www.cff.org.

Cystic Fibrosis Foundation, "Sweat Testing," www.cff.org.

Cystic Fibrosis Foundation, "Teacher's Guide," www.cff.org.

Zoe A. Davis, M.S., P.N.P., R.N., "Cystic Fibrosis," *Nurseweek.com,* May 7, 2002. www.nurseweek.com

Howard Hughes Medical Institute, "Stalking a Lethal Gene: Finding the Faulty Gene's Fellow Travelers," 2002. www.hhmi.org.

David Lott, "K-State, KU Develop Cystic Fibrosis Treatment," *Kansas State University Collegian,* June 9, 1997. www.kstate collegian.com

Mayo Clinic.com, "What Is Cystic Fibrosis?" 2002. www.mayo clinic.com

Merritt McKinney, "Study Raises Possibility of New Cystic Fibrosis Type," Reuters Health, www.nlm.nih.gov.

Pulmonology Channel, "Cystic Fibrosis," 2001. www.pulmono logychannel.com.

Websites

Howard Hughes Medical Institute (www.hhmi.org). Provides a good introduction to the genetics of cystic fibrosis.

Index

Picture Credits

Cover photo: © Simon Fraser/Photo Researchers, Inc.
© Nogues Alain/CORBIS SYTMA, 77
© Annie Griffiths Belt/CORBIS, 26
© Lester V. Bergman/CORIBS, 27
© Bettmann/CORBIS, 14, 40
© Cadwell-Gill/Custom Medical Stock Photo, 30
© JL Carson/Custom Medical Stock Photo, 70
© Jacques N. Chenet/Woodfin Camp & Associates, 47
Jeff Di Matteo, 16, 19, 37, 67
© Mauro Fermariello/Photo Researchers, Inc., 59
© Simon Fraser/Photo Researchers, Inc., 43, 44, 52, 56
© Simon Fraser/RVI, Newcastle-upon-Tyne/Photo
    Researchers, Inc., 9, 63, 74
© Logical Images/Custom Medical Stock Photo, 17
© LWA-Stephen Welstead/CORBIS, 48
© Photo Researchers, Inc., 32
© Royalty-Free/CORBIS, 60
© Howard Sochurek/CORBIS, 28
© R. Wehr/Custom Medical Stock Photo, 20

About the Author

Melissa Abramovitz grew up in San Diego, California, and developed an interest in medical topics as a teenager. She began college with the intention of becoming a doctor, but later switched majors and graduated summa cum laude from the University of California, San Diego, with a degree in psychology in 1976.

She launched her career as a writer in 1986 to allow her to be an at-home mom when her two children were small, realized she had found her niche, and continues to freelance regularly for a variety of magazines and educational book publishers. In her sixteen years as a freelancer she has published hundreds of nonfiction articles and numerous short stories, poems, and books for children, teenagers, and adults. Many of her works are on medical topics.

At the present time she lives in San Luis Obispo, California, with her husband and two college-aged sons.